Fitness, Performance
and the Female Equestrian

Fitness, Performance
and the
Female Equestrian

Mary D. Midkiff

To Karen, Coty and Bo —

Best wishes in all of your
equestrian pursuits together.

Mary D. Midkiff

Howell Book House
New York

All photographs in chapters 2, 3, 5, and 6 by Rich Frasier unless otherwise noted. All photographs in chapter 4 by Alix Coleman unless otherwise noted.

Howell Book House
A Simon & Schuster Macmillan Company
1633 Broadway
New York, NY 10019

MACMILLAN is a registered trademark of Macmillan, Inc.

Library of Congress Cataloging-in-Publication Data
Midkiff, Mary D.
Fitness, performance and the female equestrian / Mary D. Midkiff.
        p. cm.
        Includes index.
ISBN 0-87605-945-0
1. Horsemanship—Health aspects. 2. Physical fitness for women.
I. Title.
RC1220.H67M53 1996
613.7' 045' 088798—dc20   96-22537
                                    CIP

Design by Amy Peppler Adams—designLab, Seattle

Manufactured in the United States of America

10 9 8 7 6 5 4 3 2 1

To TLA from MDMA

Contents

Foreword

This book is an important guide for women who want to feel well, ride well, and extend their active years. You can learn about the female body, and specifically how to enhance your performance on horseback through a better knowledge of fitness, nutrition, and use of special techniques and equipment.

My personal interest in learning more about fitness and nutrition for riding developed as a result of my return to the competitive show jumping arena after a fifteen-year absence. I had always been an active, athletic individual and considered myself to be in pretty good shape from playing tennis twice a week and riding on weekends.

However, when faced with the more rigorous daily training and schooling sessions required for preparing a show jumper for competition, I discovered I was not as muscularly or aerobically fit as I had thought. Minor aches and pains frequently developed after intensive schooling sessions, and at one of my first competitions I was actually in an exhausted anaerobic state following completion of a particularly long, demanding jumper course.

This marked an interesting turning point in my riding career. All of my life I had ridden to get fit, but now at middle age I was going to have to get fit to ride. I located a physical fitness trainer and embarked on a program of strengthening my body. The rewards are well worth the effort. Not only am I able to ride or foxhunt for several hours without experiencing any muscle fatigue, I also have a firmer body, higher energy level, and sharper mental reactions.

This improved condition did not result from exercise alone, but from a complete program of exercise, diet, and nutrition. Most women associate those words with an unpleasant regime and do not want to be bothered with altering their lifestyle. In reality, attaining better fitness and health is not that difficult and requires only minor alterations in the female rider's program.

Most important is the commitment to a better body for life. For women, weight training is especially vital as it also strengthens bones, which can help retard osteoporosis. With the increased interest in fitness in today's society, it is now much easier to locate a gym or fitness trainer in your area. Coupled with the advice in this book, you can develop a program that will enhance your riding.

Convenient scheduling is critical to success in a fitness program. I found that having a trainer come to my house three mornings a week at 7:00 A.M. worked best for me. Of course, it required buying the necessary weight-training equipment, but I knew it was the only way to fit workouts into my busy schedule. Whether day or evening, find the best time in your schedule and then stick with it. I even take written programs with me when I travel and continue my workouts in hotel exercise rooms or local gyms.

Stretching and massage therapy are also extremely beneficial to my personal program. I have found that muscle groups must be properly stretched prior to exertion to avoid injury and provide greater flexibility. The session with my massage therapist noticeably reduces lactic acid buildup and the associated pain in active muscles. The chapters on stretching and strengthening provide you with important information on these subjects to help you, and your horse, perform better.

Dieting is something we would all like to avoid, and fad diets are to be avoided. Proper nutrition, on the other hand, is really a matter of developing sensible eating habits, and knowing which foods can actually enhance performance or help the body in recovery. In the chapter on nutrition, you will learn how to eat properly to sustain your energy levels and improve performance overall. I have found that in addition to understanding food values, an athlete must also follow a weight-maintenance program by limiting the daily intake of fat. A fat gram counter can be invaluable to women who want to lose weight or are struggling to maintain a specific weight.

Nutritional supplements can provide additional benefits in your program and are worth researching. I had been told by numerous doctors over the years that a multivitamin was not needed as long as I ate a balanced diet. But, who really eats a balanced diet? I usually fall short of the recommended levels of fruit, vegetables, and fiber. After years of experimentation on and off supplements, I have finally developed a supplemental regime that includes antioxidants and double-chelated minerals that provide me with maximum benefits and proper absorption. I have more energy and feel much better.

Once you have made exercise, body maintenance, and nutrition a part of your dietary routine, it becomes very easy to stay on a lifetime program of well-being, which will provide you with the enjoyment of riding to the best of your ability.

CHRYSTINE JONES TAUBER
International Rider
International Judge and Course Designer

Introduction

hrough my lifelong experiences with horses and horse-people, and my Women & Horses workshops nationwide, I have become certain of one thing: *Women have a special magic with horses.*

There is a natural affinity between women and horses, something so basic it creates an immediate foundation for a relationship and a launching pad for almost everything we want to do with a horse. We are passionate about horses; they sense it. We have a natural advantage in working with them, not unlike the bond between mother and child that operates through good times and bad, complicated tasks and easy ones.

Unless there is something in the mental makeup of the specific horse (or the particular human) that gets in the way, the foundation is automatic. It is there to be cultivated and put to good use. Otherwise it can just go to waste.

This book is all about three things:

1. *Insights* into the relationship of women and horses.

2. *Understanding* yourself, your horse and your horse activities.

3. *Methods* to bring out the best in you and your horse.

Not everything in this book is exclusive to women. There is plenty here for every horseperson to learn and use. The essence is female, since the themes are drawn from an understanding of why the female-horse relationship is unique, what drives it and how we can use this understanding to maximize horse-human experience and performance. The methods and techniques themselves often are less gender specific: *all* riders can gain immeasurably from recognizing what it is about the relationship that works and what elements of it can best be put to use by any individual in any specific situation.

Nonetheless, this book is undeniably female in character and the conversation that goes on throughout it assumes a female audience.

There is no need to apologize for this. In fact, the numbers associated with horse activities in North America suggest that thinking and writing specifically about the woman's role with horses is long overdue. Grassroots riding programs nationwide are full of little girls learning to ride and adult women returning to it.

Recreational horse activities and sport riding are now largely dominated by young and adult women. From backyard horsekeeping and training through Olympic-level and top rodeo competition, women have become the predominant participants and the key economic force in the horse world. If you think about it, there is good reason for this. Equestrian activities collectively represent one of the very few sports in which women compete on equal terms with men. The horse is the equalizer. The horse compensates for the inherent disparities in strength between men and women and puts the "game" on a different field. That field promotes qualities and traits in which women can excel, such as finesse, touch and understanding. This in no way disparages the competitiveness of women. Properly channeled, these capabilities translate into tremendous athletic performance by the horse-rider team (rather than the individual). And team performance is, after all, the essence of great riding.

Controlling and cultivating the effort of a half-ton animal is no small feat. Clearly sheer human strength cannot be the key. If it were, the horse would get his way every time.

The depth and breadth of female involvement carries through all levels of horse-related activity. Female equestrians represent over 80 percent of today's horse enthusiasts and participants, a fact uncovered by my company, Equestrian Resources, through contacts with the major equine breed, discipline, and sanctioning organizations in America. Interestingly, most of these organizations had not remarked upon this truth until we pointed it out to them, and more still have yet to figure out what it means and what, if anything, to do about it.*

The female equestrian is constantly balancing friendships, family, career, home and horse. One hope I have is that this book can help make the balancing act less difficult by explaining how to reduce the time and effort it takes to maximize the relationship with your horse.

Female Participation in Equestrian Organizations, 1994

Sanctioning Organizations	Total Members	Percentage Female	Total Female
American Horse Shows Assn.	60,000	81	48,600
American Quarter Horse Assn.	300,000	57	171,000
Breed Organizations			
American Morgan Horse Assn.	11,463	71	8,139
American Paint Horse Assn.	48,000	54	25,920
American Saddlebred Horse Assn.	7,360	65	4,784
American Warmblood Society	750	90	675
Appaloosa Horse Club	28,464	50	14,232
International Arabian Horse Assn.	22,637	75	16,978
Palomino Horse Breeders of America	10,815	55	5,948
Other Organizations			
United States Dressage Federation	38,000	95	36,100
U.S. Combined Training Assn.	10,662	65	6,930
Women's Pro Rodeo Assn.	1,670	100	1,670
American Vaulting Association	650	80	520
Nat'l Steeplechase & Hunt (Jockeys)	127	29	37

*In addition to the numbers involved, the demographic characteristics of this group are compelling. The research gathered from our Women & Horses (W&H) Workshops nationwide indicates the most predominant female, thirty to thirty-five to forty-five years of age, humanities college education, and participates in dressage or recreational riding. She is active, dedicated and has expendable leisure income. Her horse is the center of her recreational life.

Female Participation in Equestrian Organizations, 1994 (cont.)

Sanctioning Organizations	Total Members	Percentage Female	Total Female
American Endurance Ride Conf.	5,000	76	3,800
The Carriage Association of America	3,500	40	1,400
Youth Organizations/Division			
United States Pony Clubs	12,931	90	11,638
National 4-H (Equine)	240,143	69	165,699
Intercollegiate Horse Show Assn.	4,500	93	4,185

AWAREness

I have tried to condense our insights and methods into a stream of "awareness" issues that run through the text. The acronym AWARE (A Woman's Approach to Riding Effectively) appears throughout to signal these key summary points.

Most of us have been taught which buttons to push with little understanding of what is going on with our bodies or our horses. The purpose of AWARE is to give female equestrians information about their physical attributes, fitness, health and nutritional considerations and issues that surround her and her horse. For example, my contributors and I give you insight into the dynamics of the female anatomy and how it works with the movement of the horse. You will learn what tools to use at home, in the barn or at an event to make your body and mind work more effectively with your horse. The key is to establish the *connection* between the insight (why) and the method (how) to put it to use.

Ultimately, AWAREness is about giving female riders a basis of understanding that stems from what comes naturally to her. Between the lines, you will find the answers to questions many of us share but have been too embarrassed to pursue.

AWAREness. Use this book as a resource. It has been purposely designed to be just that. I have included a number of historical references for you to better understand how women have evolved in riding. Some of the quotations are laughable and hard to believe in the context of today's (supposedly) progressive world; others have stood the test of time remarkably well and remain relevant to what we are experiencing in the modern world.

This is an all-discipline, all-breed approach to the female's riding issues and concerns. Keep in mind, however, that we are all individuals and there are exceptions to all rules.

Especially as they apply to women.

And horses.

Chapter 1

What's behind the Magic

The sight of that pony did something to me I've never quite been able to explain. He was more than tremendous strength and speed and beauty of motion. He set me dreaming.—Walt Morey

y their nature, horses are passive grazers, living and moving in herds. In the wild, they are hunted and stalked by their enemies. Their instinctual response to fear or the unknown is fight, flight, or freeze. If you've been around horses much, you've seen them react in this manner to various environmental changes, as well as in their socializing with other horses. "Like all herbivorous creatures that love to roam in herds," wrote Elizabeth Karr in 1884 in *The American Horsewoman*, "the horse is naturally of a restless temperament. Activity is the delight of his existence, and when left to nature and a free life, he is seldom quiet."

If you transfer these natural behavior patterns into a domestic training environment, you will see them show through in the way the horse responds to the handler and trainer. If the horse is uncertain of the trainer's intentions, or is introduced to something new, or is unclear about the message, or is in pain, it may run away, freeze up or fight. Think about how you've seen horses respond to fear or pain. Did they hide in the corner and sulk, or come at you with all four hooves, flat ears and a threatening mouthful of teeth? In any given instance, the horse may duck out, bolt, buck, bite, strike out in front or a combination of all of these in a fraction of a second. These are the horse's

1

natural response mechanisms at work. They are designed for protection and survival.

Add to this circumstance of nature a set of human-based considerations. We are generally associated with the rules that govern a horse's existence, many of which it may rebel against or at the very least ignore. We communicate by speaking; horses do not (at least, not in a spoken language). Thus, to a horse we convey our intentions, affections and other communications in tangible actions that are often accompanied by sounds to be associated with those actions.

Given this set of facts, step back and think about the kind of person who would work best with a horse. Chances are you've begun to think in terms of a gentle touch, a soft but firm voice, an intuitive sense of the factors triggering a behavior, a calming effect, sensitivity instead of force and a constant search for more meaningful communication with the animal. This description certainly fits the human female. Women want to tame, save and nurture the beast. (To a fault—just look at some of the people we marry.)

Why We Love Horses and Why They Love Us Back

"Women value love, communication, beauty and relationships," says John Gray in *Men Are from Mars, Women Are from Venus*. "They spend a lot of time supporting, helping and nurturing one another. Their sense of self is defined through their feelings and the quality of their relationships." The public television program *Men, Women: The Sex Difference* notes that humans have had four million years of gender training. Women are gatherers, nurturers and teachers, while men are proficient at spatial tasks and hunting for survival. Women have spent most of their time through history teaching and caring for the young. They have an innate ability to read emotions, learned basically by reading a baby's cues without language. It all adds up to "woman's intuition," not the abstract concept typically referred to in wonderment and awe, but rather a very real ability to understand and predict based on behavior. Most of us have it, even if we haven't consciously used it or have allowed it to slip into disuse.

These female traits carry into the horse world and translate into positive behaviors and messages that can allow the horse to be more relaxed and more trusting, and ultimately to perform to its potential. After all, our relationship with horses is one of our most cherished, and they feel it through the positive and loving energy coming from us.

One of the most compelling reasons women love horses is the promise and reality of unconditional love. Horses give much and expect little in return. They can be the proverbial big, cuddly teddy bears who also happen to be able to run like the wind. They are beautiful, spirited, elusive animals that nuzzle us and cajole us. They capture our interest and feed our curiosity. The affection with which we treat them usually comes back in kind, like human children (before they get the keys to the car). When we've had a bad day, when we want to be alone, or when we've got news to share, our horses are always there for us.

AWAREness

Horses communicate through behavior, so they look for signals from you through your behavior. Your actions—the way you do things—are much more important than the meanings of words you use.

I've seen the connection to human child-rearing repeatedly through personal experience and workshops around the country. Through their horses, women with grown children seem to recapture some of the lost elements of their mother-child relationships, particularly the gratification associated with teaching; women with young children are constantly commenting on the similarities and differences between their human and horse "kids"; and women who are without children for whatever reason often appear to vent some of their displaced or unutilized nurturing on the animal, whether they realize it or not.

Without resorting to amateur psychoanalysis, it is clear to me that the horse fits easily into the learned nurturing model of the human female—perhaps even the nurturing *ideal*, since you can put the animal away in a stall when you get tired or its behavior gets out of hand (all of this, plus the sheer joy of riding, exercise, fresh air and interaction with other women who share the interest). Not a bad deal.

Although today we prefer cooperation rather than domination, horses reward us for good treatment and care. Unlike people, they live in the present and don't calculate or manipulate. They respond with signs of pleasure, happiness and relaxation, and reflect the kindness back with a genuine welcome when we arrive on the scene.

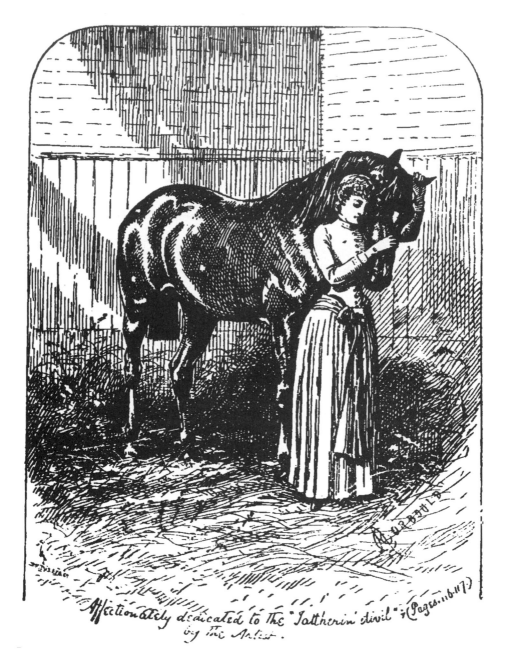

"To the mistress who thoroughly understands the art of managing (horses), the horse gives his entire affection and obedience, becomes her most willing slave, submits to all her whims, and is proud and happy under her rule." —The American Horsewoman, 1884.

Horses make us feel good. That reward alone can make our day and relieve stress. At our Women & Horses workshops we hear about the special relationship between women and horses:

> As a female I want to make a connection with horses rather than dominate them.
>
> Horses are the perfect children: They don't talk back.

Even a century ago, the connection was evident to Elizabeth Karr: "In disposition the horse is much like a child. Both are governed by kindness combined with firmness; both meet indifference with indifference, but return tenfold in love and obedience any care or affection that is bestowed upon them."

Both women and horses are social animals. Women enjoy socializing, sharing problems and successes with other women much more than men do with other men. Women love to talk, especially to each other. Horses are the vehicle. A barn environment becomes a "country club." What's more, a horse lends itself to being groomed, dressed up, shown off and talked about.

That's why we love them and they love us.

That's what's behind the magic.

A Brief History of Women Riding

There isn't much documentation by or about women and their riding. We do know that women have been involved with horses since the domestication of the animal some six thousand years ago.

The issue of riding sidesaddle versus riding astride has commanded much attention as something of a bellwether in the history of female equitation. It is commonly assumed that women rode sidesaddle until the modern era, but the facts don't support it. In 1932, a significant change was noted and put in its proper historical context by authors Diane Shedden and Lady Apsley in their book *To Whom the Goddess*:

> Thirty years ago, women riding other than sideways in England could almost be counted on the fingers of the two hands, while now the numbers must be fairly equal so that the cross-saddle [astride] seat is often referred to as 'the modern,' and the women who do so as 'new fashioned.' But as a matter of fact the earliest women riders rode astride.

It is on record that a Roman general commanding the army occupying the Rhine in the days of one of the later Emperors was reprimanded for riding in trousers and permitting his wife to do so also (trousers, of course, being the garb of Barbarians and as surprising to the Romans as a general hunting in a kilt would be to us today!). In fact, all women who rode at all, rode either astride or pillion behind a man till the fourteenth century. The first side-saddle is said to have been introduced into England by Anne of Bohemia, wife of Richard II, about 1380, but for a long time side-saddles were only used by the wealthiest of ladies of quality; for the majority it must have been a matter of astride or pillion-riding. A Dutch print of 1572-1619 shows a woman riding sideways in a pannier saddle with a foot-rest on a palfrey with bad shoulders, decorated with a plume of feathers on his bridle, while an etching of about the same period (1600) shows a lady riding astride in baggy breeches tied over the knees by ribbon garters finished by large bows. Some fifty years later evidently both seats were in vogue. Hortense Mancini, the attractive Duchesse de Mazarin, ran away from her dull husband, scandalizing everyone by riding across Europe dressed 'in Cavalier costume,' and took refuge with Charles II in England.

Today a woman may please herself entirely as to which seat she adopts without upsetting anyone, and she should weigh the pros and cons of her particular case as she is best suited.

The authors point out that "all women who rode at all rode either astride or pillion behind a man till the fourteenth century." The sidesaddle came into vogue after that.

From as early as the seventeenth century, the eastern parts of the United States and Europe considered a "woman's saddle" a sidesaddle. Women rode sidesaddle because it was not proper or acceptable for a woman to spread her legs and show her petticoats. It was also uncomfortable to ride astride without underpants, pantaloons or boots. Societal mores determined women's dress of the early 1700s on and off the horse. Volumes of petticoats under a full skirt; a high collared blouse; a fitted vest with top coat; a hat adorned with flowers, feathers or ribbon; gloves; and shoes and stockings completed every "proper" woman's attire when she went out.

Europe set the standards in the 18th century, and the colonies were eager to emulate the "mother country." Upper-class women would ride recreationally by dressing

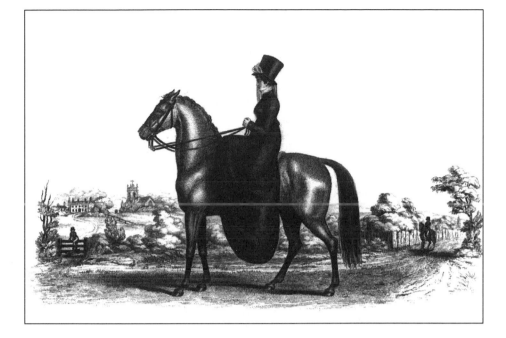

Proper woman's riding attire in the 1700s. Credit: The National Sporting Library.

up and saddling up a favorite horse. This was often the only time when women could comfortably gossip or discuss delicate issues not to be aired in mixed company. The horse provided an escape and became a symbol of freedom from societal constraints and family pressures. (Sound familiar?)

A woman was typically "in the increasing way" throughout her childbearing years (that period accounting for more than 50 percent of her lifespan), making it more difficult and uncomfortable to ride often. And even when she did ride, sitting the trot in a sidesaddle (without a leaping horn) for hours was not exactly pleasant. Falling off was a common occurrence—hardly something to look forward to—and trying to get back on an even greater challenge.

In the United States, even runaway female slaves only found it acceptable to ride in a "woman's saddle."

The 1850s saw the introduction of the leaping horn, also known as a pommel, leaping-head or curved crutch (an apparatus on the sidesaddle for support of the right leg; *leaping* was the term for "jumping"). This change made riding accessible to many more women. It gave them confidence over fences by providing greater balance. Hunting with men became more attractive; divided skirts, boots and pantaloons came into fashion. Some women even began to ride astride in a "man's saddle" (the forward seat saddle of today) in the hunt field.

"In these days of 'advanced' ideas the advisability of women aping man in yet another way, by riding astride, is the subject of general discussion," wrote Belle Beach in her 1912 textbook *Riding and Driving for Women*. "Many 'authorities' upon riding—'mere men,' it is needless to say—speak with enthusiasm of the day when all women will ride in this, for most of them, ungainly and unbecoming fashion. Personally, I deplore the tendency and believe that it is a mere passing fad and that, except under peculiar conditions which I shall mention, most women ride best and look best in the side-saddle."

On the frontier, however, women did what they had to do to survive. "The Western Girl learned to take her place in the saddle and often behind the trenches with her brother," says Marnie Francis Hafley, a National Cowgirl Hall of Famer. Women grew up in the saddle and took charge of the homestead, with the children and livestock as their companions. Even if a woman were married, her husband was not around often. She never knew when or if he would return from hunting or surveying. Moving cattle, driving wagons, plowing and daily chores involved horses. So while her cousins in the East lived by fashion codes, the frontier women lived by survival necessity. Horses meant survival.

"Some women tried to pass as men by wearing men's clothes and binding their breasts. They could get along more comfortably, felt safe and could accomplish more. Especially for riding, getting by as a man seemed more practical and healthier in the long run," says Virginia Artho, assistant director at the National Cowgirl Hall of Fame in Hereford, Texas.

Groups would get together and form rodeos and competitions. Some of the "wilder" women became involved in traveling Wild West shows and rodeos, presenting their horses and themselves as entertainment.

Saddle design was advancing, too. According to Beach in 1912: "In the west the Mexican type of saddle is generally used. This saddle has a high pommel, or even a high horn in front and a very high cantle serving as a back rest, making what is practically a 'dished out' seat, far

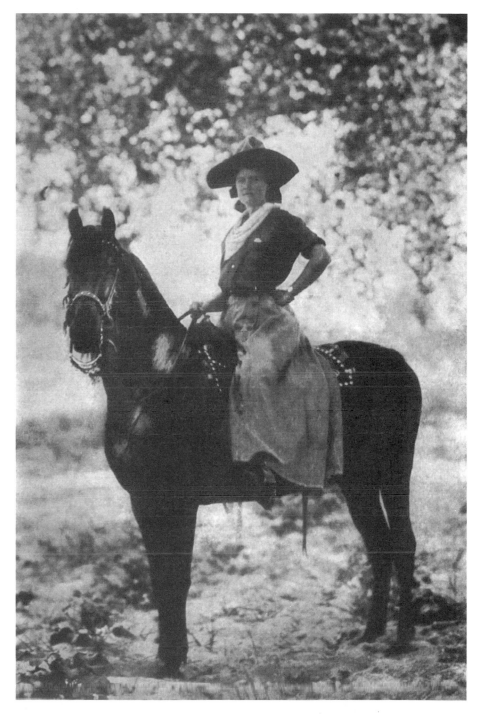

Typical Mexican or Western riding attire and gear for women in the late 1800s. Photo: The National Sporting Library.

better suited to a woman's conformation than the English saddle."

Evolution and Revolution in Riding

At the advent of the Industrial Revolution with its motorized machinery and transportation, the identity of the horse as a worker began to fade. America was sending its first equestrian team to the Olympics in 1912, marking the advance of horses beyond racing, work and the military, and recognizing them for their recreational and sport abilities. (The first female equestrian team member to represent the United States was Marjorie Haines in 1952. She competed in dressage and placed seventeenth overall as an individual. The U.S. team placed sixth.) One constant was that people used the animals as status symbols, as they still do today. On London's Rotten Row, women and men showed off their best riding habits and mounts to each other, competing for attention. Some women competed in horse shows and wore breeches and boots like the military-trained male competitors. Women in America's major East Coast cities were doing the same. If it was fashionable in London and Paris, it was the height of fashion in America's growing cities.

The mechanizing of the cavalry in the 1950s permanently changed riding (and the future of the horse) in America and set the stage for increased participation by women. Suddenly, the government owned thousands of domestic riding horses, well trained and ready for action.

Mrs. F. H. Prince, Jr. "leaping" sidesaddle, 1948. Photo by Thomas Darling, courtesy of Howard Allen.

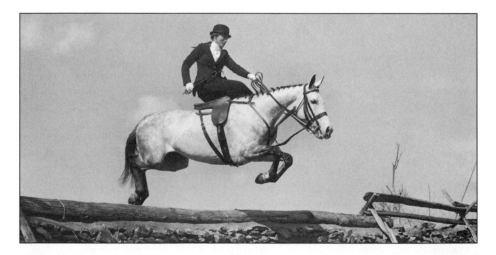

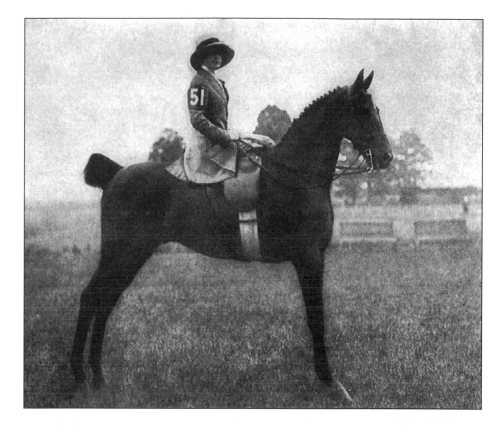

*Kentucky-bred
ladies' saddle
horse, c. 1910.*
Photo: The
National
Sporting
Library.

Through disbursements, auctions and sales, many of these horses moved on to recreational and show careers. Light-horse breeding, as distinct from the production of heavier draft types, began to grow, with many of the foundation mares and stallions coming from the cavalry units. "Designer horses" started to appear, created more and more for specialized use and increasingly suited to the female equestrian. Breed associations began marketing to the rec-reational user and the novice rider and encouraging their breeders to focus on the amateur and part-timer rather than the professional.

Meanwhile, from the 1940s onward Hollywood played on women's romantic notions about horses with *National Velvet* and *Nautical*, *Black Beauty* and *My Friend Flicka*, *Fury* and even Mr. Ed. Glamorous stars rode astride on the big screen and later on television.

More versatile horses found a welcoming partner as the sexual revolution gained strength through the 1960s and women became increasingly independent. With more personal income and reliable birth control, women became empowered to fulfill their lives as they wished, and their connection with horses advanced. We women had always loved horses; now we were increasingly free to enjoy them on our own terms.

Modern Times

Riding traditionally has been strongly *task oriented*, relating more to the job at hand than developing the skill of the horse. Since men did most of the relevant tasks, they did most of the riding and training. Horses were used for transportation and work on farms. There were certain jobs that soldiers and cowboys had to accomplish every day with their horses. Look to Europe to see how men used horses to obtain food (pure sport came later). The most prolific history of the horse comes, of course, from the battlefield, which was dominated by men.

Today, however, we use horses for fun, as entertainment and as a recreational outlet. In North America, horses do not exist out of necessity for human survival. Horses are in the latter stages of reinventing themselves (unknowingly) as a vehicle for our entertainment, sport and pleasure—an adaptation that is saving them from extinction. Without the work-based identity of the past, they exist increasingly because people, particularly women, simply enjoy riding, driving, being around and looking at them. Otherwise, they would be an endangered species.

AWAREness

The emancipation of both women and horses has taken place in the 20th century.

The big news is that the days of male domination of riding are gone. Our equestrian traditions may stem from a work ethic and the male point of view, but that no longer fits with today's realities. The female element is increasingly defining and directing modern horse sport and recreation. Just ask any tack store owner what percentage of customers are women. The natural affiliation of women and horses has found a happy home within our modern societal trends. "Many women today are tired of giving," author John Gray observes. "They want time off. Time to explore being themselves. Time to care about themselves first. As a woman matures she also learns new strategies for giving, but her major change tends to be learning to set limits in order to receive what she wants."

What we want is a horse.

In the United States today, hundreds of thousands of women and girls spend after-work hours and weekends with their horses. We get together on the show circuits, with friends from a barn or riding club for a trail ride and lunch, or at home for a horse video party. We may not remember each other's names, but we remember each other's horses' names. Most female equestrians would rather spend time cleaning the barn than their own house.

This female equestrian phenomenon appears to be more pervasive in the United States than in other countries, although Germany is beginning to see a shift—two-thirds of the German Equestrian Federation's membership is female. Men and women share horse sports almost equally in Europe. From my perspective, this is both because of the number of American women involved (because of the socioeconomic changes described above) *and* the relatively sharp decline in male participation in the United States. America isn't as tied to tradition as Ireland, Great Britain and other European nations where the horse sports, originated thousands of years ago, were and in many cases still are male-dominated.

While most men are involved in other sports in the U.S., women have found a meaningful and competitive outlet with their horses. In August 1994, *Advertising Age* reported that "Swimming and golf top the charts as the most popular adult sporting activities, according to a survey from Simmons Market Research Bureau, New York. Men enjoy participating in softball/baseball much more than the general population, while women are more likely to be horseback riders."

It is time for awareness and instruction to accommodate this reality, and with it the female rider's specific issues and needs.

Chapter 2

The Female Rider *Is* Different

with Mary Beth Walsh, P.T.

. . . The necessity for prescribing rules to which the young Horse-woman may occasionally refer, in order to guard against falling into certain errors which are at all times attended with a degree of danger, induces the Author to submit this brief work to the Public, which he flatters himself will be found greatly to assist Ladies in the acquirement of a sufficient knowledge of Riding for the common purposes of exercise, which, he humbly conceives, is as much as is necessary for them to acquire in the art; as, from the peculiarity of their seat, they must not expect to arrive at any great degree of proficiency in the higher airs.—Edward Stanley, *The Young Horsewomen's Compendium of the Modern Art of Riding,* 1827

*E*dward Stanley figured that all the education in the world would not be enough to overcome the peculiarity of our seats. Well, at least he noticed that there is a physical difference between men and women. Unfortunately, his skepticism over the ability of the female rider lurks in many corners, even today.

Formal English riding instruction, which stems from the days of the military and the hunt field, traditionally has been biased toward the male rider, his body type and physical strength. Western riding stems from life on the ranch and the range, historically biased toward the male rider, his body type and physical strength.

That has left a gap in some very basic understandings about how women's issues relate to riding, as well as problems with the equipment and techniques associated with managing and performing with the animal. For instance, how many riders and instructors realize that women's hormonal changes can relate to their joints and threshold of pain? During the middle of the menstrual cycle as well as a few days prior, we experience an increased level of the hormone estrogen which lowers a woman's tolerance to pain. Therefore, we experience more aches and pains, particularly in our joints at this time. Some women may even complain that they feel their joints are more "lax," however, research in this area has not proven this to be true.

———
AWAREness
Understand your
body first.
———

This is not an excuse or a rationalization for reduced effort. There are days when a woman simply can't put a "leg on" as effectively, due to physiology and her cycle. Understanding this can make life a lot easier for both the rider and the instructor. Maybe it's a good idea to take it easy and hack out instead of jumping a course or working on lateral movements during that time. Injuries and a great deal of frustration can be avoided, along with the horse's confusion about it all, with increased awareness of your normal body cycles.

Do you believe that women (and not just women riders) can be more productive if they understand their anatomy and body type? Do you know how the specific physiological and psychological issues associated with being a woman can impact your riding? Do you know that there is equipment on the market made specifically for the female rider? Do all instructors know about this equipment and how it can improve performance? Or, for that matter, why equipment is made for the female rider in the first place? The answer to each of these questions needs to be "yes" before we can hope to maximize our performance and enjoyment with horses. What's more, it is up to us to articulate our issues and share them with our instructors and others involved in our riding. They can't read minds. (Not yet, anyway!)

To get us started, let's meet Mary Beth Walsh, an invaluable resource, a friend and one of our Women & Horses Workshop and National Tour experts. Mary Beth is a physical therapist on the faculty in the Physical Therapy program at Marymount University in Arlington, Virginia.

She has combined her British Horse Society Assistant Instructor Certification and experience as a physical therapist to work on women riders' physical issues, along with non-riding concerns. Her physical therapy practice is located in northern Virginia, and it specializes in the back and neck. It is currently almost exclusively sports medicine–related. She has implemented an equestrian rehabilitation program into her everyday practice and lectures on related topics through the Women & Horses Workshop tours.

Using Mary Beth's wealth of knowledge and practical experience, let's look at the physiology of the human female and why it makes a difference in your riding. If the going gets a little technical for your taste, don't worry: We just want you to understand some basic points about how you are built and what you need to do because of it. The goal is to understand your own body type, identifying the areas of individual strength and weakness, and sharing this knowledge with your instructor and/or trainer, whether male or female. (Communicating your specific issues is vital.)

Once again, remind yourself that riding is not about strength. It's about balance, flexibility, good body awareness and communication. These are all qualities that women can develop and refine. As a woman, you have a built-in set of advantages in getting your horse to respond to you. We know that women generally have less strength and muscle mass than men, and we have learned to compensate with technique. Women are natural "finesse" riders. We use our minds, calculated movement and resourcefulness before resorting to strength. (A friend of mine who is a fly fishing instructor makes a similar observation, noting that women often make better fly fishers because they "finesse" the rod and line to gain a long cast, whereas men who are learning the art typically try to "muscle it" and in so doing lose a lot of distance—but perhaps gain a little humility and some appre-ciation for "touch.")

Nonetheless, the physical differences between men and women play a role, and we have to recognize and deal with those differences before we can get on to refining our innate capabilities.

At the most basic of levels, men and women come in all different shapes and sizes. There is a fundamental difference between the two: Women are essentially pear-shaped. We have a wider base at our hips, with most of our muscle mass and strength in our legs and pelvis. Women have a smaller shoulder complex, with less muscle mass and strength in the upper body. Because of the distribution of muscle mass and body shape, women have a slightly lower center of gravity than men, which provides for a better base of balance.

Understanding your body type and your natural propensities will help you recognize your natural strengths and focus you on aspects of your body that require special attention. Humans generally fall into three basic body types:

- The *mesomorph,* the most common body type, is essentially a muscular build that can carry some extra weight. Mesomorphs tend to be athletic.

- The *ectomorph* is thin and lanky, like a ballet dancer or distance runner, and the type we see most often in dressage. Ectomorphs have long lean limbs, but generally suffer from some degree of inflexibility and have to concentrate on stretching to compensate for their long extremities.

- The *endomorph* is a more rounded body type with a lower proportion of lean muscle mass and a greater propensity for being overweight. With correct training, the endomorph can increase lean muscle mass toward that of a mesomorph. This body is typical of the person who is quite fit but carries some extra weight, such as football and rugby players, shot putters and discus throwers.

The significance of the specific anatomic difference between men and women extends from the basic shape of our body frames to the way we use our bodies (the shape dictating certain abilities or shortcomings), and ultimately to the way we ride a horse. Although men, due to their anatomy and pelvic structure, have the ability to find and maintain a "deep seat" or "tucked" seat underneath themselves with little effort, women have the advantage with a lower center of gravity providing them with more security in the saddle. Men are more top heavy and must work hard to avoid "teetering around," whereas women must develop their upper bodies to complement their lower base. It naturally follows that men and women logically may have to follow different paths (or techniques) in order to get the same result on a horse; we have to do different things to compensate for physiological differences. If we don't, then one of us is going to end up sore, injured or just plain frustrated. Until now, that usually has meant women, since riding techniques and equipment were almost entirely geared toward men.

A more specific area of physical difference between men and women centers in the pelvic complex (which includes the sacroiliac joint, pelvic bones and hip joints). You might assume that women have larger hips than men because we tend to be more pear-shaped, and you might further assume that this is so because we have a bigger pelvis to accommodate giving birth. However, on examination of male

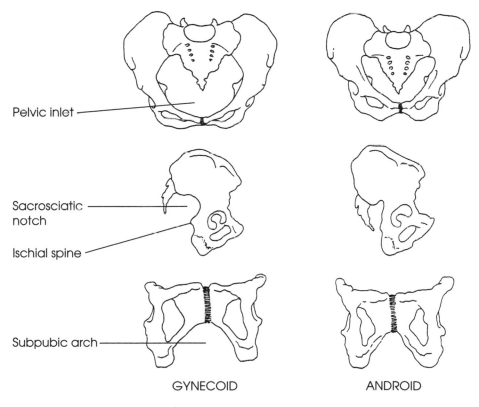

GYNECOID   ANDROID

Three views of the female (left) and male (right) pelvis. Reprinted by permission from David J. Magee, *Orthopedic Physical Assessment,* 2d ed. Philadelphia: W. B. Saunders Company, 1992.

and female skeletons, we see that it is the *shape* of the pelvic bones that differs, not the overall size of the hips. Notice that in the diagram comparing the male and female pelvis, the "fork," or the pubic ramus, differs in shape—the male's is more angular while the female's is more oval and rounded. This allows for a larger channel in the center of the pelvic complex, which serves as the birth canal in women.

Also notice the angle of the sacrum, the triangular-shaped bone that forms the posterior aspect of the pelvic complex. The sacrum in the male tends to be tilted back, causing a flattened angle at the joint with the lumbar spine. In women, the sacrum is tilted forward, creating an increased curve at the juncture of the lower back. The result: In riding, this pelvic configuration causes the male to ride with his pelvis underneath him, with a slightly flattened back. In women, the tilt of the pelvis promotes a tendency to ride with more weight on the "fork" of the seat (somewhat arched in the back). The correct seat, male or female, is that of *balance* between the two extremes. More on this in chapter 4.

————
AWAREness
Men and women have to take different routes to the same goal.
————

Spinal alignment is also crucial to the woman's riding posture and balance, as the illustrations on page 25 show. The rider in the slouched position has a flattened curve that causes a C-shape throughout the spine. This posture puts strain on the ligaments of the back, causing the shoulders to round and the head to protrude forward. At the other extreme, the rider with the arched back limits the motion of the lower back by "jamming" the lumbar spine. This position puts unnecessary weight on the fork of the seat, which leads to pain, abrasion and saddle sores. The ideal position for any rider, male or female, is to locate an "in-balance" position evenly over both seat bones with a gentle, supple curve in the lower back (see page 26). This allows the pelvic complex to move with the horse's movement. This position also promotes good alignment throughout the spine and down through the hip and leg.

The orientation of the hip bones in the hip socket also presents a male-female distinction and, therefore, has an effect on riding. This orientation dictates how the leg will

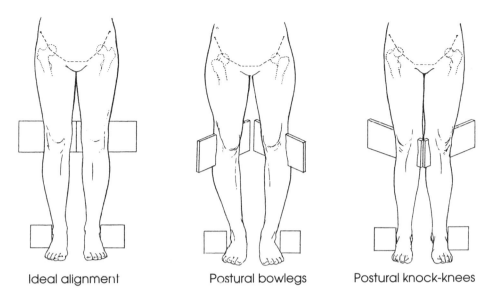

Ideal alignment   Postural bowlegs   Postural knock-knees

Three examples of hip bone orientation seen in women. Reprinted by permission from Florence Kendall et al., *Muscle Testing and Function,* 4th ed. Baltimore: Williams & Wilkins, 1983.

be positioned under the body. Look at the illustration above. The internally (medially) rotated position causes a bow-legged position that is common in males. (That problem is addressed in chapter 6 with a series of stretches and exercises.) Conversely, the externally (laterally) rotated position causes the thighs to approximate each other, creating a knock-kneed position much more common in females. The implication for riders is obvious when you think about it: If the angle of the hip causes the legs to be pressed together, it simply makes getting the legs around the broad barrel of a horse more of a strain. This leads us directly to an important adjustment for the female rider: We have to emphasize stretching the inner thigh, hamstrings and quadriceps that surround the pelvis.

The angle of the hip also affects how the quadriceps, the muscles of the anterior (front of the) thigh, attach into the knee. Many women suffer from anterior knee pain. The primary cause is the acute angle of the knee, which places undue pressure on the inner portion of the knee. Symptoms of this phenomenon are discussed along with other rider concerns in chapter 5, "Common Injuries and Their Causes."

Female Anatomy 101: Putting the Parts Together

The female rider sits astride the horse in the same align-ment that she would stand: with her feet spread wide apart and her knees slightly bent, heels roughly aligned with shoulders. In the saddle, the major difference, of course, is that the base of support is no longer solely in the feet (excuse the pun); the weight is distributed throughout the inner leg and thigh, with the center of balance being the seat bones (the ischial tuberosities) and the fork of the seat (the pubic ramus).

Think of your skeleton as a series of building blocks stacked in progression. Every bone in your body is con-nected to another bone, so what moves or affects one joint of the body will also have an effect on another joint. This is known as a *closed chain reaction*. Familiar examples of closed chain reactions mounted are: (1) Mouth of horse connected to rider's hands through the reins; or (2) when we are in the saddle or riding bareback we are connected to the horse through our seat and legs. All the forces that affect the seat are also going to affect the joints further up the body. Recognizing these connections is extremely important to the rider. For a quick lesson in anatomy, we will start with the backbone and work our way up the spine and out to the periphery.

The *spine* is made up of a column of thirty-three bones called vertebrae. These vertebrae are stacked one on top of another in an S-shape. The *spinal column* seats the skull or cranium at the top and connects the hip bones or pelvis at the base. The spine curves, forming an inward arch (lor-dosis) toward the top, an outward one (kyphosis) toward the middle and another lordosis at the bottom, or lumbar spine. The spine houses the nervous system and the spinal cord, which is actually an extension of the brain, with nerve roots extending from each vertebral level. These nerve roots act as an electrical system, dispersing information from the brain to tell our bodies what to do and relaying messages back to the brain to transfer what we are feeling, such as pain or motion.

In between each pair of vertebrae is the intervertebral disc. The *disc* is a unique joint in that it is composed of rings of soft cartilage and encases a jelly-like substance, thus allowing fluid movement in many directions and a degree

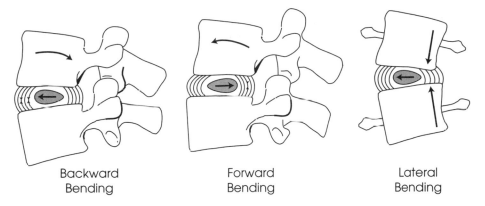

| Backward Bending | Forward Bending | Lateral Bending |

Effects of backward, forward and side bending on the inner part of the disc. The biomechanics of the disc are very much like those of a jelly donut. Adapted from Kapandji; reprinted by permission from H. Duane Saunders, *Evaluation, Treatment and Prevention of Musculoskeletal Disorders.* Minneapolis: Anderburg-Lund Company, 1986.

of shock absorption. The biomechanics of the disc are much like those of a jelly donut; if you compress one end of the donut, the jelly gets pushed to the opposite side. If you repeatedly push on one side of the donut, the jelly eventually erupts from it. When a similar condition occurs in humans, it is called a herniated disc. Herniated discs are most often caused by repeated forward bending motions, "slouching" or poor lifting techniques. The prevention of this problem is crucial to riders because of the constant bending and picking up associated with riding and barn work.

The bony joints of the spine, called the facet joints, are aligned to act as rails to guide the movement of the spine in some directions and to prohibit movement in other directions. See the illustration on page 27 that shows how intimately connected all the structures of the spinal column are.

The S-shaped curve of the spine is necessary to distribute the forces of the body equally and architecturally. It is easier to maintain this type of structure in an upright fashion, as opposed to a stick-straight object or a C-shaped structure. The gently curved spine is particularly important when we look at correct equitation and the mechanics of riding.

The curves of the spine are primarily maintained with two major ligaments (ligaments attach bone to bone, tendons attach muscle to bone). The two major ligaments running in the front of the spine are broad and thick, like those of a horse; the ligament in the back part of the spine is narrower and thinner. Some paleontologists theorize that humans once moved in a quadruped, or all-fours, position like horses, dogs and apes, necessitating this kind of structure. Since we have more support in the front part of the spine and less in the back, we stretch the weaker ligaments every time we bend over or slouch.

Ligaments are not the only source of support for the spine. Muscles of the trunk, including the spinal extensors that initiate the backward bending of the spine, the spinal flexors or abdominals, and the muscles of the shoulder and the hip also affect it. The relationship of these muscles is discussed further in chapter 6.

The *pelvis* attaches to the spine at the sacrum, the fused portion of the vertebrae. The pelvis is actually three separate bones—the sacrum, ilium and ischium. The seat bones are actually part of the ischium, while the fork of the seat is the ilium, which makes up what are called the pubic bones. These bones are not connected by ordinary joints but are bound tightly together by many ligaments. These ligaments may stretch with a hormonal stimulus, such as pregnancy. For example, during pregnancy and labor, joints will become more lax and stretch somewhat to allow passage of the baby through the birth canal. These bones can also shift with severe trauma (like a hard fall) directly onto the pelvis. The actual hip bone is the attachment of the thigh bone (femur) to the ischium. (See pelvis comparisons on page 150.)

The *hip joint* is a ball-and-socket joint, and allows movement in four planes of motion—side to side, up and down, and in and out. Thanks to immense ligament and muscular involvement, it is a very secure joint. This entire structure is very different in males.

The *shoulder* girdle attaches from the level of the sixth cervical vertebra, with the collarbone (clavicle) in the front and the shoulder blade (scapula) in the back.

The *arm bone* (humerus) forms with the shoulder a ball-and-socket joint, enabling movement in many directions. Due to the mobility of the shoulder joint and the lack of muscle development in many women, it is particularly vulnerable to strain and dislocation.

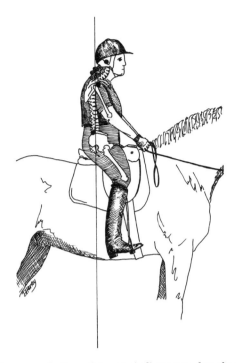

Rider slouched. Notice how severely the neck is out of alignment when the chin and head are leading.

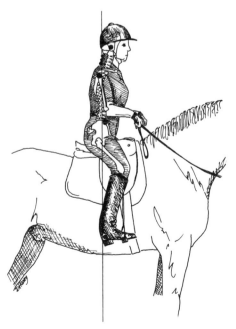

Rider with arched back. There is no connection between body parts, and the spine is not able to absorb concussion.

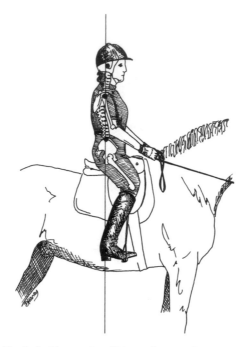

Rider "in balance." The rider looks like a series of hinges that can function together.

Now that we have a frame of reference, let's discuss what makes these old bones move: the *muscles*.

All the muscles work together in some form of synergy, or movement pattern. Functionally, no muscle works alone to make a body part move. Essentially, one opposing muscle group must contract as the other muscle relaxes. For example, as we kick our leg out, our quadriceps on the top of the leg contracts as our hamstring on the underside relaxes.

Though greatly oversimplified, this does essentially demonstrate how most muscle groups work.

AWAREness

Understanding the differences in the female hip joint and how your body works while mounted are instrumental to success in the saddle.

The second way muscles work together is to co-contract, or work simultaneously around a joint to stabilize it. The best example of this is in the spine. To correctly support the spine, the spinal extensors must contract to maintain the body upright while the spinal flexors, or abdominals, also contract to stabilize the front part of the body and control the tilt of the pelvis. This forms a natural "corset" to keep the spine upright.

The third way muscles work together is to stabilize one part of a joint to act as a fulcrum so that another muscle group can work more effectively. For example, when we raise our arms up over our head as in a chopping motion, muscles that hold the shoulder blade in place stabilize the shoulder blade so that the deltoid, or front muscle of the shoulder, can lift our arms more effectively. The rotator cuff muscles of the shoulder distract the arm bone from the joint to a certain degree as we raise our arm over our head to prevent jamming in the joint as this motion occurs.

You can see that body movement requires the cooperation and interplay of many muscles and joints. Any weakness, tightness or injury in any particular muscle group can

Rear view of the major muscle groups and the spine of a mounted rider.

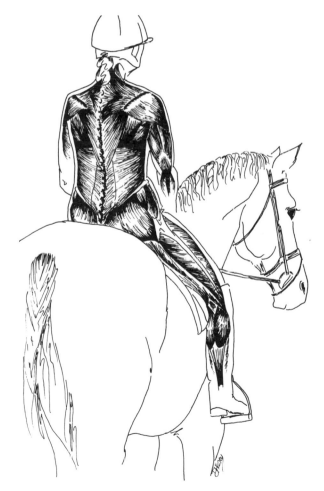

affect the function of another. That's why minor injuries can turn into major problems.

Understanding how all these muscles work and being aware of how your body works in riding (and more specifically, in certain types of riding) is crucial in training, both in the saddle and in your fitness program. The previous illustration shows the major muscle groups and how they function.

Now that you understand the basics of movement, let's see how these bones and muscles interact with forces generated by the horse when you ride it.

Chapter 3

Let the Force Move You

The rhythm of the ride carried them on and on, and she knew that the horse was as eager as she, as much in love with the speed and air and freedom. —Georgess McHargue

*R*elaxation, comfort, and effectiveness. These are the three key results of understanding the biomechanics of riding, or how your body works with the horse.

Any riding activity is what is referred to biomechanically as a *closed chain activity*. This means the limbs of the body as well as the seat are in contact with an object, and all the forces that impact the most peripheral joint affect every joint farther along the body. This chain effect is caused by impact on a surface, referred to as a ground reaction force.

When we walk on our own two feet, the ground reaction forces start when our heel hits the ground, our foot flattens to absorb the shock of impact, and we push off with the ball of the foot. The force of heel strike, how well we absorb the impact and how effectively our muscles push off will affect the foot, ankle, knee, hip and lower back. If we have a problem in our foot, such as fallen or high arches, it will change the reaction of forces throughout this chain and cause trauma to multiple joints and muscles. That is why many people wear arch supports or orthotics in their shoes.

The Human-Horse Connection

When we ride, we add a few more forces in addition to the ground. Our feet are in contact with a stirrup, creating one chain; our seat and leg are in contact with the horse, a second chain; and our hands are in contact with the horse's mouth or head via the reins, creating a third chain.

Riding is a unique closed chain activity because the ground reaction forces impacting the rider are generated by the ground reaction forces moving up through the horse. Every step a horse takes sends a reaction up through the rider. Thus, the type of gait a horse uses directly influences the rider. For example, if the horse has a short choppy trot, those vertical forces will be translated to the rider; conversely, if the horse has a nice sloping shoulder, a long pastern and a smooth shock-absorbing gait, the vertical forces will be reduced.

A horse's walking or trotting gait emulates that of a human. That is one of the many reasons horses are used in therapy for the handicapped. The movement of the walk promotes forward propulsion; reciprocal motion of the legs follows, causing rotation through the trunk and a weight shift from side to side. In other words, the horse helps "teach" the body of the handicapped rider how to walk.

When a horse trots, as when a human jogs, there is also an upward transference of movement. The canter of the horse is unique in that it has (or should have) a three-beat pattern, pushing off with a hind leg, then landing in sequence with the other legs, creating a "rocking" motion. The faster the gait, the greater the forward propulsion and upward translation. Thus, during a gallop, it is easier to raise yourself off the horse's back, which in turn frees up the motion of the animal's back and its hind legs. This explains why jockeys stand in the stirrups almost the entire time they are mounted. The only time they are seated is generally during the post parade, before the race, at the walk. If they were seated at a gallop during the race, it would impede the motion of both rider and horse, and the jockey would most likely never forget the bumpy ride.

Understanding the forces of the gait of the horse is very important in developing the ability to "go with the movement of the horse." In chapter 4, Peggy Cummings suggests using a small trampoline to gain a better understanding of this movement and to train yourself to accept and transport the motion through your body. Our intention here is to prepare you by explaining what joints and muscles need to be flexible and strong before you get in the saddle, so that you will be able to have a comfortable and effective seat and aids.

Body Mechanics

When riding, the *seat* is composed of the two seat bones and the fork of the seat. The seat also extends down the leg equally on both sides of the horse via the hip joint, alongside the inner thigh and leg. The movable joints of the seat are the lumbar (lower) vertebrae and the hip joint. When the horse is moving, the forward, upward and rotational movements have to be absorbed through the lumbar spine. This is accomplished with the pelvic tilt type of motion.

This is a forward-and-backward motion of the hips, controlled by the lower abdominals, which pull the pelvis backward (like pulling your seat underneath you) to flatten the lumbar lordosis. This is followed by a controlled relaxation of the abdominals, allowing the pelvis to tilt forward and increasing the lumbar lordosis (arching the back—like a duck).

When we sit upright, our back muscles, or spinal extensors, are always contracting; otherwise we would roll up in a heap. To maximize our effectiveness in the saddle, we must constantly be aware of controlling our abdominal contractions, especially if we don't already have good muscle tone in this area. The pelvis also rocks from side to side as the horse shifts his weight with a little rotation. The upward forces of the movement need to be absorbed by moving in sync with the horse, while keeping the joints and muscles relaxed. It is much more likely for a sack of potatoes to move, settle and balance than it is for a sack of bricks. The muscles and joints can absorb shock better when they are relaxed.

The hip joint is a very important part of the pelvic complex. It allows the pelvis to rock forward and back. Sitting astride, our hips are in a separated position. In

---

AWAREness

The key factor with the pelvis is to learn to allow the horse to move you and your hinges. Don't try and force it or imitate the tilt motion to stay in sync. "Appearing" still while the horse is moving requires a great deal of motion in our bodies.

females, there is a strong tendency for the hip to turn in, or internally rotate, in the toe-in position, the much-maligned "running like a girl." Picture for a moment a woman running with her knees together and her feet turning outward. (If you've seen an old Jerry Lewis movie lately, you can picture what this looks like in the extreme.)

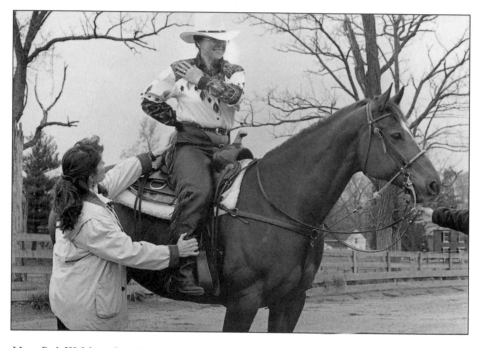

Mary Beth Walsh works with trainer and instructor Alice Magaha on hip and leg flexibility and shows her how it can affect her entire body.

To be the most effective in your riding, the leg should be turned inward, or internally rotated at the hip. Women may have to work a little harder to master this position. The muscles of the front part of the hip, the quadriceps and iliopsoas, need to be supple in order to place the leg in line with the pelvis. The hamstrings and gluteus maximus on the back part of the hip need to be supple to allow the gentle curve of the lower back to exist. Look at the next illustration to understand how leg muscle inflexibility affects the lower back and hip and, ultimately, the ability to move the pelvis as necessary for a good supple seat.

Think of the last time you yanked your leg back to achieve the correct position, only to find that your pelvis

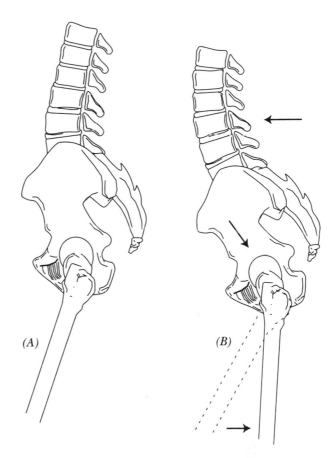

(A) *Hip in a correct, flexed position with a soft lower back. (B) The lower back tends to arch when the leg is pulled too far back. You lose hip flexion, maximum seat contact and body mobility.* Reprinted with permission from George Davies and James Gould, *Orthopaedic and Sports Physical Therapy,* 2d ed. St. Louis: C.V. Mosby Company, 1990. Adapted from A. Steindler, *Kinesiology of the Human Body under Normal and Pathological Conditions.* Springfield, Ill.: Charles C. Thomas, 1955.

rocked forward and your lower back arched. This phenomenon is known as *relative flexibility.* When one joint along the chain is tight, as shown in the illustration, the joint above or below it will accommodate the motion to achieve the desired movement. If we do not correct the stiffness in one joint, overuse will occur at the more supple joint. This is one of the many causes of lower back injuries in female riders.

The other important muscle group of the seat is the inner thigh muscles. These muscles comprise the adductor muscle group that pulls the legs together. In riding, these are often referred to as the "gripper" muscles; novices often try to stay in the saddle by using them to squeeze the horse. This actually has an adverse effect—the contraction of these muscles holds the seat away from the horse, preventing a relaxed and deep seat. The same occurs if these muscles are tight, which keeps our legs from draping comfortably around the horse. One of the chief causes of muscle soreness after riding, particularly if you haven't ridden in a while, results from sitting in a position of stretch for a prolonged period of time, or perhaps gripping with the adductor muscles.

—•—

AWAREness

Relaxed muscles and joints are better shock absorbers than tense ones.

—•—

The *two-point position* requires that we rise out of the saddle, in which case the base of support is solely through the leg. This is a closed chain activity, with our feet in the stirrups and all the muscles of the leg contracting and working. Here, the knee and ankle must be supple and relaxed, absorbing the up-and-down motions during the rising trot and in the two-point position. The calf muscles (gastrocnemius and soleus) are crucial for allowing gentle shock absorption to occur. If the heel is jammed down and fixed in place, it stops the chain's flow through the joints, eliminating the vital shock-absorbing action. This is not supple, comfortable or effective.

Research has found that the muscles of the leg (namely the quadriceps and the gastrocnemius) are the best shock absorbers, as they allow controlled bending, or flexion, in the knee and ankle to accommodate movement. If these muscles are tight or fixed, as they are when your heels are jammed down, the next joint to absorb the shock is the lower back, which is not designed to withstand constant concussive forces. One of the best presentations of the right way to do it that I've ever seen comes from Olympic Gold Medalist Nicole Uphoff-Becker, whose thighs and pelvis absorb the motion and move with it instead of pushing against it. She seems still, but there is a great deal of motion "inside" her joints.

The chain of the body continues through the shoulder-to-hand complex. Good alignment—the head in line over the shoulder and the shoulder in line with the hip—is critical for optimum function of the arms. The forward shoulder and jutted-out head posture assumed by many riders is caused by weak muscles in the scapulae and shoulders. It is also caused by poor postural habits when you're not riding. It inhibits the normal function of the shoulder by limiting the range of motion and placing the strong stabilizing muscles of the shoulder at a biomechanical disadvantage.

Simply put, they can't do the job because you're putting your body in a position that makes it impossible. When the shoulder is forward, it cannot glide back and forth naturally to move with the forward and backward motion of the horse's head on the flat, or by releasing effectively over a fence. This also disrupts the correct line from the elbow through the hand to the rein. As a result, the follow-through movement occurs at the elbow or wrist, creating an unnatural and ineffective aid.

To maximize our riding, we need to strengthen the muscles that support the shoulder: the trapezius, rhomboids, serratus anterior and latissimus dorsi. Shoulder weakness leads to poor control of the hand, as well as poor alignment in all aspects of riding (especially while maintaining a "folded" position over a fence).

We strengthen our muscles so that we can be stronger—but not "harder"—in the saddle. We concentrate on relaxation and flexibility in order to work with the horse and protect ourselves. In sum, we work with, not against, the natural force. We let it move us (and our horse).

Female biomechanics and the forces generated by riding should now be coupled in your mind, creating a general awareness of what is happening when you sit on a horse. Now let's get a lesson in riding technique designed for (and by) women.

Chapter 4

More Performance with Less Effort

with Peggy Cummings

Women are turning to horses not only for pleasure and sport, but for a way of reducing stress in their lives. "What do you want from riding?" is one of the first questions I ask in my clinics all of the time. Regardless of discipline or level, the answers are always the same: to have fun, improve my riding, have a good partnership with my horse, be safe, with less pain or discomfort.—Peggy Cummings

Learning how to use your body to support and enhance the movement of the horse is what Peggy Cummings' work and this chapter are all about. Unwittingly, many of us get in the way of our horse's ability to perform and move. As female riders, we are often unaware of how our bodies can communicate "mixed messages" that realize ineffective outcomes.

Do you believe you can achieve performance purely with balance and finesse? Are you sure that you are "allowing" your horse to reach its full potential in movement and performance? You probably can identify with compression (stress) in your life, but can you identify compression in your riding? Think about those questions for a moment.

No matter what the level or discipline of horse and rider, a female rider's body must be able to respond and go with the motion of the horse in order to convey clear messages and intentions, redirect movement and get results. Peggy Cummings teaches how to allow and convey those clear messages. As I've gotten to know her, I've come to admire her real talent as a "horse and rider communication specialist." And being the mother of six children, she certainly can identify with our female-specific body and lifestyle issues.

Peggy Cummings is an internationally respected instructor and trainer. She travels throughout the country instructing and training riders involved in all breeds and disciplines. She has thoroughly researched her craft through years of experience in riding, beginning with her childhood in El Salvador, her teaching Pony Club and at girls' camps in Maine, running her own teaching and training barn in Maine for seventeen years, receiving her Horsemaster's Certification in Maryland and instructing in Pennsylvania from 1990 to 1994. Her home base today is in Hailey, Idaho. She travels extensively, conducting clinics and training sessions.

Peggy is also a Master Centered Riding Instructor and a TT.E.A.M. (Tellington Touch Equine Awareness Method) practitioner. She has combined her classical background and years of working with noted experts to establish her own methods and techniques. Peggy's motto—"Motion is the means, freedom of movement is the outcome"—says a great deal about her philosophy of riding and life. You have to keep moving to achieve true freedom in your riding and in your life. Her talents also extend to human body work, where she has studied acupressure and is currently involved in Alexander Technique training.

From the very first time we got together, what Peggy conveyed to me made sense. She understood my specific issues right away, as a woman and as a rider, and at the same time did not invalidate my years of training and teaching. She broadened my horizons and gave me new resources. I've heard the same comments from many others as well.

We've had experiences at our Women & Horses workshops with riders who for reasons of their own—including injury and fear—have determined that they would have to cut back on or stop riding. After hearing and working with us, that outlook changed. They possessed a new level of comfort and optimism based on the new tools they had been given. That is the essence of Peggy's work and the essence of this chapter.

As of this writing, one of our mutual friends is competing at the Grand Prix level in dressage abroad, hoping someday to make the Olympic team. She has told me repeatedly that she would not be riding Grand Prix at all if she hadn't worked with Peggy to develop awareness and movement in her body to accomplish the tasks required at that level. And what about those of us who are stuck in our bodies at First Level? The stories I can relate about Peggy's positive influence on riders are endless.

All female riders can benefit from an awareness of their body and how it works with the movement of the horse. The preceding chapters have set the stage for putting a basic understanding of the female body together with the motion of the horse in order to produce better results. And now, through Peggy, we can learn about and understand how to achieve more with less effort and discomfort. As women, we have to resolve our physical issues before we can fully accomplish goals with our horses.

What follows has been compiled after observing Peggy's work at clinics and workshops and through interviews with her.

Women Are Searching for Other Ways to Work with Their Horses

In light of all of the financial, emotional and physical commitments and investments we have in our horse(s), it is amazing that women keep riding "in spite of" pain, discomfort, fear and frustration. With regard to the horses, it is equally amazing that they serve us "in spite of" the way they are ridden, cared for and treated. This says a great deal about the essential bond we have with our horses, our mutual goal to keep trying to make things work well "in spite of" whatever comes along. We have been taught to believe and expect that, as with many sports and physical activities, no pain means no gain. Is this the optimal approach to riding? We challenge this "norm" and see it as counterproductive to effective riding.

Much of the riding being taught today derives from times and approaches that are no longer appropriate or relevant to our riding needs. There are many and varied reasons historically for the ways riding has evolved. Many techniques made sense in their time. Cavalrymen and cow-boys, for example, had very specific tasks at hand and a certain amount of awareness and knowledge available with which to work. The job descriptions for horses and riders have changed dramatically, yet our methods of riding, train-ing and caring for horses have not changed to meet the needs and demands of the new jobs. Until now.

The traditional ways we have been taught equitation include "sit up, sit still, push down, pull back, squeeze, show him who's boss and kick with both legs." Dominance and force are still the primary modes in working with horses. There are still many trainers using side reins, draw reins, gag and twisted-wire bits and other contraptions, along with fear tactics to get results because they lack the knowledge to do it any other way.

And it isn't only outmoded, force-based riding that cre-ates resistance in our horses. Improper nutrition, poor shoe-ing or unbalanced feet, and ill-fitting tack and equipment are contributors as well. Both horse and rider react to pain in the same way—they shut down, or resist, in order to pro-tect the affected area. Over time they become locked in their protective stance.

We, as well as the horses, pay the price for a lack of knowledge and patience. The heartening thing I find as I travel around the country is that women in particular (but not exclusively) are searching for other ways to work with their horses.

Less Is More

When we are at our wits' end in a particular situation, the tendency is to resort to more leg, more hardware (such as severe bits, martingales, draw reins, riggings, etc.) and more work and effort. Paradoxically, less is more. Every time Peggy teaches her students—novices to advanced riders—how to realign their positions and allow motion in their bodies, they feel better and their horses relax and lengthen their strides. The horses begin thinking instead of reacting and are able to become partners instead of disobedient or evasive beings.

AWAREness

Finesse rather than force is the only approach that makes sense.

At one of her clinics, Peggy measured horses' stride lengths and compared them when the riders were in balance and out of balance. The out-of-balance riders were those who rode with a tight, arched back or with a saggy back and collapsed chest. The shortest stride lengths recorded were from the riders with arched backs, followed by the saggy-backed riders. The horses with balanced riders consistently had the longest stride lengths. This area deserves more research and it certainly raises questions about the effects of the rider's position and tension in her body on the horse's performance.

Riding with more awareness and less effort by allowing natural motion in the human body creates positive outcomes. There's no magic or voodoo involved. You simply capture the forces of motion and let them help you move ahead, rather than react to them as unwanted byproducts of the activity. This is a basic, logical, commonsense approach, and it works with all types, breeds and disciplines.

This knowledge can help you find a well-matched horse with comparable physical attributes to fit your body. It can help identify a horse with the best conformation to perform in the discipline you want. And it leads the way to understanding equipment, such as a properly fitted saddle, which is basic to success with any horse.

Sending Messages

When you use your aids or "send a message" to your horse, what happens? Peggy asked about sending messages in her clinics, and women around the country responded with these comments and observations.

- The horse evades, resists or ignores what I'm asking for.

- What works with one horse doesn't always work with another.

- What the instructor suggests isn't working for me or the horse.

- There's an impasse at learning a particular movement—I can't find a point of reference to break through

- Changes in my body (due to injury, aging, stiffness, etc.) are making it harder for me to communicate.

Do these sound familiar?

We all have varying degrees of tightness or rigid places in our bodies, as well as right- or left-sidedness. These potential limitations in the rider's body send restrictive messages to comparable places in the horse's body. Many riders lose sight of or don't recognize the impact their own tight bodies and predispositions have on the performance of the horse.

Many women have been following instructions for years without really feeling what those instructions mean to them or the horse. It's just accepted as the right thing to do because that's the way it's been done. Each rider translates commands—more leg, hold him back, use your seat, get your heels down, half halt, sit up and put your shoulders back—differently. These lessons are filtered through your personal history with horses: injuries or fears, successes and failures, body awareness. Or maybe we just never learned to feel the right response from the horse, or understand why we did or didn't get what we asked for.

As Mary Beth Walsh mentioned earlier, the "closed chain" means that one action begets a series of reactions down the line. In addition to your direct messages, your body actions send indirect messages as well. Add ill-fitting equipment effects on top of that, and we have a substantial set of information pieces that our horses interpret and react to. These contribute to the imbalance of the horse.

AWAREness

A horse can feel a fly on its back, so you can just imagine what a tight human body feels like. This is why horses can become either hypersensitive or insensitive to the rider's aids.

Confusing Commands

Were you ever told you were too weak or unfit to be a good rider? Have you ever been asked for "more" and you don't know how you could possibly give "more"? How many times have you been told you need more leg, more upper-body strength, and muscle power to get the job done?

Interpreting your equitation instruction is a personal issue built on all sorts of personal conditions. Many of the commands we are given in riding instruction can be confusing, scrambled messages. We hear them and react to them by guessing at what the instructor wants. Nobody explained the function. Alternatively, we don't do it because we just can't do it; our body gets so tight and tense, it just can't move.

Following is a list of typical commands in a riding lesson and how they are usually handled or "interpreted" by

---

The Vicious Cycle: English Example

Many horses get called names such as lazy, sour, hyper, spooky, etc., when in reality the horse is reacting to tightness in the human body.

We make many choices for our horses. In addition to deciding the direction the team is headed in and the moves we're going to make along the way, we also make tangible decisions about things like equipment. Mistakes in the process can trigger a series of unwanted results.

Improper saddle placement, for example, triggers a cycle of problems that result in an out-of-balance condition. When the saddle is placed forward onto the withers, it impedes the motion of the shoulder blade at each stride, and severely affects the horse's ability to rebalance itself. Basically, the horse is being forced onto its forehand because the constriction of the saddle and the forward weight of the rider puts it there.

The "heels down" position also prevents the ankle, knee and hip joints from responding to the movement of the horse, thereby locking the leg and acting as a brake or brace against the forward motion of the horse. It's like driving with the brakes on.

Arching the back acts much the same way. This stiff spine becomes a jackhammer, directly pounding into the horse's spine. The rigidity of the rider's body in this position actually creates the feeling of "dead weight" to a horse's back. It is like carrying a load of bricks: heavy and immovable. This position then creates a horse that is forced onto its forehand, stuck in the withers, and thrown off balance by a rider who is unable to go with the motion. It is virtually impossible for the horse and rider to find rhythm and balance in this position.

Chronic physical problems can result from this scenario. For the rider, it may result in joint pain with sore knees. For the horse, always on the forehand in this situation, it may result in front-end problems such as lameness, navicular, above or behind the bit, falling in or out, lack of forward movement or constant jigging. The horse is put in a position of being constantly out of balance with no way to recover. Evasions are built on this kind of foundation.

The Vicious Cycle: Western Example

Western saddles are often cut too big or too long for a particular horse's conformation, and subsequently misplaced on the back. This can cause stress and irritation to the hips, which leads eventually to hind-end soreness, front-end problems, irritability and tension in the horse.

Many western riders put their "feet on the dashboard," placing the feet and legs forward. This position puts their upper body behind the motion of the horse. It is not uncommon, particularly with men, to find them in a more slump-backed position, with the lower back and chest being held in a collapsed position.

Here, the rider is always trying to catch up to the motion of the horse instead of staying in balance. The horse will either respond by becoming more nervous and anxious or else dead-sided, ignoring your aids. These are evasions due to imbalance.

---

the rider. Peggy has put this list together from years of observation and experience in body work. These are some examples of what happens to the body when you act out the command.

1. More Leg, More Leg

The notion of "more leg" usually implies pressing with your legs around the horse's barrel. This ends up being compressive and static, a "dead signal." Clamping on with the leg does not send a clear signal to move. He may move with this signal but it will be a reaction to "get away," not "work with" the rider. By clamping, tension is created through the lower back, which inevitably causes rigidity in the upper leg; the pressure of the lower leg becomes static and less effective. Rigidity adds to loss of power and rhythm. All the "hinges" or joints in the lower half of your body stop moving and flexing. How does your horse react to this signal to supposedly "go" when your body is saying "stop"?

Try it on a friend. Have your friend get down on all fours. Straddle her and clamp your legs against her waist. Ask her what it feels like. Now try it again with a soft "released" back (see page 54) and a slight walking-forward motion, or while vibrating alternate legs against her waist. Does she feel more encouraged to move on?

2. Sit Up and Pull Your Shoulders Back

"Sit up and pull your shoulders back" creates a tight and hollow lower back and restricts the rider's breathing ability. These restrictions put you behind the motion of the horse. It also restricts the natural alternating movement of the arms and makes a light following hand impossible to achieve. So while the object here is to look good and maintain an erect posture, you are causing your horse to stiffen in the front end and drop or tighten the back. Another mixed message for both of you.

3. Push Your Heels Down

Pushing the "heels down" in an attempt to become more secure restricts the flexibility of all of the joints and pushes the leg forward. The ankle joint is stiffened when the heel is pressed or jammed down. You are supposedly trying to stay more secure, but in reality, the more rigid your body is the less stable you are, and you are less in synchrony with the movement of the horse's body.

4. Use Your Seat

"Use your seat" often finds the rider tightening the buttocks and lower back to create the effort of "use." If you are balanced and flexible, there is no need to tighten or flex any muscles to achieve the desired effect. Your tight back and buttocks will be reflected in a shortened stride and less "push" from behind in the horse.

5. Keep Your Hands Still; Sit Still

When the hands are still, that is, lacking movement, they become a brace or a wall for the horse's mouth to bump or set against. There is no connection or following. Why not say and think "let your hands feel lighter and more elastic."

"Sit still" to many of us means, freeze—don't move— become a statue. When we receive this command, we immediately become rigid and problems begin. The goal is to be one with your horse; learn to follow and re-balance with his movement and you will appear "still."

All of these commands may be interpreted through the individual's filters, but they have the same effect—driving with the brakes on. Our goal is to send the horse clear messages for forward impulsion, and our bodies should be saying the same thing.

If you get a chance to watch a horse race sometime, notice how jockeys pull up their horses after the event. Have you noticed how they brace their bodies against the horse with locked elbows, locked straight knees and jammed-down heels, and lean backwards? He or she is putting on the emergency brakes to slow down a freight train. Some of the best jockeys at the top of the game don't lock up and do "allow" the horse to come back into balance with them. Julie Krone is the best I've seen in changing this typical traditional position, which over time is as tough on the horse as it is on the jockey's body. Even when a horse is being tough with her, she flexes, bends and stays soft. She weighs under 110 pounds and can finesse a one-thousand-pound colt going full speed.

Jockeys can accomplish more by changing their bodies, and we can too. We as recreational, show and sport riders are basically doing the same thing as the jockeys, only in a more subtle manner with slower or less motion and impulsion. The joints must hinge and flex for the horse to balance and work with us as a partner.

Horses work against us when we are locked or fixed. These evasions of the horse are a result of loss of the rider's balance. Understanding the impact of the motion of the rider's body on the horse is the key to improving communication and performance, particularly for the female rider.

Balancing the Body

Riding is in many ways analogous to dancing: two bodies moving together in rhythm with one person leading and providing the support and guidance to maneuver successfully. Imagine being on the dance floor with a great partner. Doesn't it feel effortless when you're moving together in sync?

What does it feel like when one or both of you are out of sync or unsure of the next move? This is comparable to what happens between horse and rider. When you apply this to dancing, it may be easier to see what really happens when one or both of the dancers falls out of sync, balance or rhythm. If you've ever experienced that feeling, you know it happens for a variety of reasons. The goal, however, is always the same: synchronization.

Everyone agrees that Fred Astaire and Ginger Rogers made it look easy. So did Olympic ice dance skaters Torville and Dean. What do they have in common with riders? The individuals and teams must learn how to rebalance themselves and their partners in a split second. Their flow appears to be flawless and almost still because there is motion in their bodies. They are experts at regaining rhythm.

It is the rider's job to be aware of the interplay of the horse's and rider's bodies in order to discern when they are in or out of balance. This is a nonverbal, kinesthetic communication. It is something that must be felt to be understood. The feeling comes from practice and awareness. It is learning to re-balance through movement. Being able to recognize the first indications of imbalance is as important as knowing when and where the balance point is found. Because riding involves continual movement of the horse and rider, rebalancing becomes the constant.

AWAREness

Being able to recognize the first indications of imbalance is as important as knowing when and where the balance point is found.

Peggy reminds her students often, "The only constant is change and the only freedom is movement." It should now be clear why static positioning of the rider creates conflict between the movement of the horse and rider. This conflict is frequently at the root of many evasions and your soreness.

The Out-of-Balance Rider

There are many symptoms or warning signs that indicate balance problems. Certainly every rider has experienced frustration from time to time when things are not in sync. However, it is the regularity of these symptoms that indicates the need to address the issues differently.

Symptoms of Being Out of Balance

Frustration and burn-out: You feel as though you can't quite get things right and you get into power struggles with the horse to get him to listen and respond. You expend a huge amount of effort in riding, with unsatisfying results. You use force and intimidation with a horse because it works.

Anne Calligan of Chester Springs, Pennsylvania, demonstrates an out-of-balance position with her arms straight, elbows locked, stirrup under her toes, leg forward, neck forward and heel pushing down.

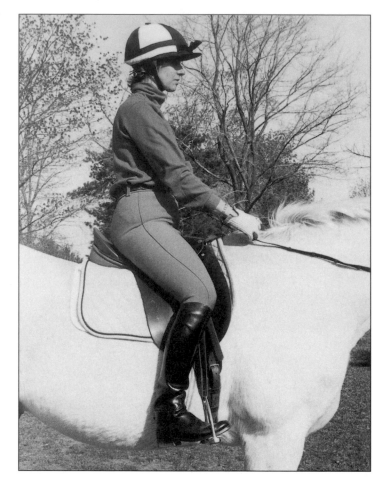

(How much is enough with an animal that outweighs us tenfold?)

This becomes an exhausting battle, one that none of us needs. Power struggles and overexertion are areas that create soreness and pain in our bodies. Women experience shoulder, neck and back pain and become more susceptible to injury when we resort to force over finesse.

Blaming the horse: Horses are sometimes blamed for things that are caused by a rider's lack of tools to effect change in the horse. You become desperate for solutions when you are unable to fix a problem with your horse. Feeling frustrated, blaming your horse or resorting to punishing yourself means it's time for outside support to help you acquire tools to rebalance the situation.

Out-of-balance rider "sitting up" with arched back, thighs tight on the saddle, heels pushed down and elbows stiff.

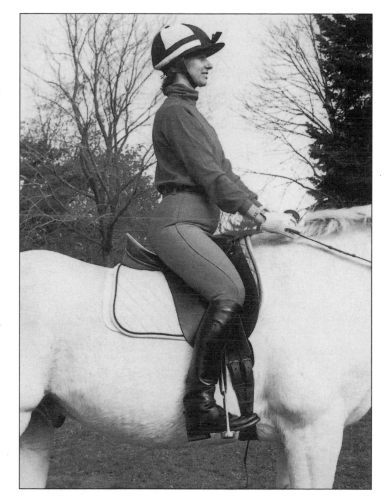

Tension and compression in your body: Riding out of balance creates tension and compression. Often this tension becomes accepted discomfort in the rider (the no pain, no gain theory) and manifests itself as muscle soreness, cramps, tight back, knee pain, chronic falls and injuries.

Have you ever had saddle sores or genital swelling and irritation? Peggy reports that most women she works with say they thought that was "just the way it is" when you ride. Think about how we compensate in our balance and position to avoid hurting ourselves further in the saddle, and the unwanted consequences are clear.

Quit because you believe riding exacerbates your soreness and pain: Back pain, neck pain, hip pain and joint pain all seem to go with the territory. Many women quit because they believe riding only makes it worse. It doesn't need to.

These symptoms are evident when the rider's body is tense and out of balance. Consider for a moment the addition of insult to injury when an imbalanced, tense body is perched on a moving object! It only leads to more tension, more insult, more injury.

Tension also has comparable effects on horses, and just as often, it too is taken as part of the deal. Chronic stocking up, anxiety in tacking up, discomfort in grooming, tripping, falling, muscular tension and discomfort are some of the results of tension and compression from the rider.

The In-Balance Rider

A majority of riders are riding behind the vertical (i.e., with the upper body tilted backward), which puts tension in both horse and rider. Women can best communicate with the horse by being biomechanically able to move freely with the natural movements of the horse's body.

Use the photograph of the in-balance rider and follow along as we go down the body. You can use this as a checklist with yourself and your friends or students.

The Peggy Cummings Checklist for the In-Balance Rider

1. **Head**   The head is centered over the shoulders with the chin parallel to the ground; the back of the neck and the jaw are soft.

2. **Upper Torso**   The upper body is free to move from the hips, allowing a buoy-like movement, which is a body's innate ability to readjust and maintain balance with the motion of the horse. (Another helpful image is of a sand-bottomed punching balloon: No matter how hard it is hit or jostled, it comes back to balance.) Breathing is also an essential part of maintaining balance. Exhalation allows the body to "catch up" with the motion and rebalance itself.

3. **Arms and Hands**   The whole arm complex is soft, above the withers, with the arms in a straight line from the bit to the elbow ready to move up or down,

forward or back with the movement of the horse's head.

4. **Elbows**   Elbows should always remain bent, soft and flexible.

5. **Lower Back**   Release the lower back and keep it full and soft. (See the section on "Release.")

6. **Seat**   Seat centered over the middle of the seat bones.

7. **Hips**   Hips should be open and centered over the seat bones.

8. **Legs**   The legs hang free out of the open hip joint.

In-balance rider with a connection from ear to shoulder to hip to heel. Use this photograph as a guide through the "in balance" checklist.

9. **Knees** There should always be bend in the knees no matter which style of riding you use. A straight knee is an ineffective hinge.

10. **Feet** The stirrup should be placed just behind the ball of the foot, allowing the joints to move. The foot is positioned parallel to the ground.

In balance in a two-point position.

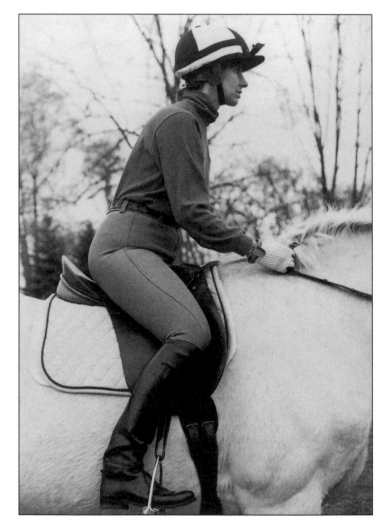

These parts complete the whole balanced position, which allows for maximum freedom of motion in the rider and, as a result, greater stride length and freedom of movement for the horse. All the hinges in the body work together to follow the motion of the horse. Even if you are in a two-point or forward position, the hip, knee and ankle are allowed to move and work together for maximum effectiveness.

Achieving Balance

Following is a series of concepts and methods to help you achieve balance in your riding.

1. Release the Back

When the spine is free of tension, it allows the upper body to lighten and rebalance naturally. It reduces the pressure on the hips, allowing them to move independently of each other; the seat bones can then follow the movement of the horse's back. The rider's legs are allowed to drape on the

To achieve balance in your position, you must first learn to release the back.

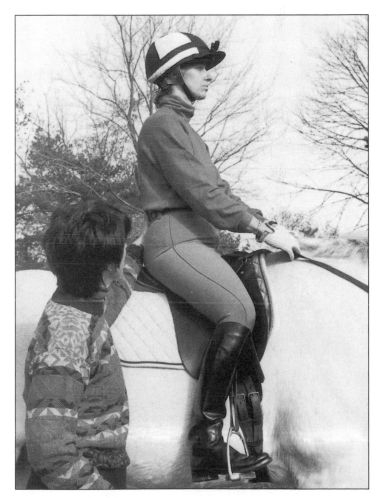

barrel of the horse, thus further allowing free movement of the knee and ankle joint. These are the signs of a released back and the beginning of synchronized riding.

"The most important message I can share with women is: Learn how to use your body with awareness. Release is the most important tool for good communication with your horse," Peggy says. Most female riders have some sort of back-related soreness. Learning to release your back is the basis for balanced, grounded, pain-free riding.

Many women who suffer from back pain are either unfit for their riding activity, overdoing it or using their body biomechanics incorrectly. Some soreness does result from lack of muscle tone and use, but as women we also have to be aware that we have to work a little harder to get our seat bones centered and our tail bone underneath us. Releasing our backs furthers this goal. Our bodies were constructed to deliver babies, first and foremost. It is easier for us to arch our backs and stay out of touch with the horse. This is an anatomical fact and it can be overcome by using exercises that increase pelvic mobility.

To Release the Back

Mounted, begin by placing your hand (or having your instructor's hand) on your back and *slowly* stroke from the shoulder blades down a few times to imprint the feel of your spine and back muscles. Now focus on the small of your back. This area is where there is a natural curve from the waist down. With your hand, sense how your back feels when you are in your normal riding position. Is there tension? Does it feel tight or rigid? Is there a deep curve? Do you arch or round your back?

The lower back cannot release unless your neck is soft and relaxed. Take a deep breath in, let the rib cage expand and feel as though air is filling into your lower back. Exhale and feel your body sink. A soft, full feeling should exist. Your back is now "released" and has settled into a flexible and relaxed mode, ready for movement.

You can learn to release your back while dismounted, too. Whether standing or sitting, try to achieve that full, soft feeling in your lower back without slumping or rounding your shoulders. Focus on your lower back as if it were a wide belt across your hips. Softening this area will naturally allow your pelvis to move.

Releasing will assist you to maximize your effort in any activity. I use it when climbing hills or hiking, vacuuming the house or lifting objects around the barn. It really saves you. Learning to release your back and using correct body mechanics is the key to injury prevention and freedom from pain.

Here are some useful exercises for achieving back release:

Knees-Up Exercise

When the knee is up in this position, the back is not arched and should not be rounded. It gives the rider a very different feeling in her back.

Drop your stirrups and place your knees together above the pommel and think about your seat bones in the saddle. Are they centered and even? Remaining in this knees-up position, place your hand in the small of your back again. Ask your instructor to feel it also. It should feel smooth, full and soft. The tension is gone.

The Knees-Up exercise will help you identify that full, soft feeling every time you get on. It is a good stretching exercise. I've also found it helps me to find the most level part of the saddle.

Back Melt

Have a friend stand behind you, with you in your familiar standing posture, and move her hand down your back and below the waist. Ask the friend to note how your back feels. Now have the friend slowly lift you up by your belt loops. Have her hold for a few seconds and then slowly let go. You should feel an immediate sense of release or melting in your lower back. Your assistant should once again move her hand slowly down your back and note the feeling. Every time we have tried this exercise, a "melting" feeling has occurred in the lower back. Keep this image in mind while you are mounted and it will help you in releasing your back. (This will not be as obvious to people who stand with a rounded back or locked knees.)

We could all benefit from an exercise in which someone leads the horse while the rider has her eyes closed and allows her body to follow the horse's motion. The feeling is very different and can produce a reawakening in one's understanding of riding.

The Knees-Up Exercise. When the knee is up in this position, the back is not arched or rounded. It gives the rider a very different feeling in her back.

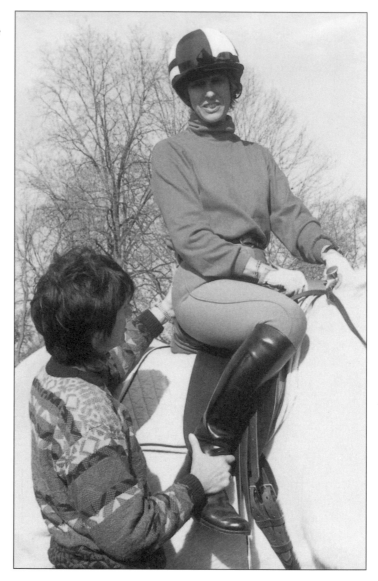

2. Use Your Legs Separately

As we've mentioned, gripping, pressing or clamping with the legs means compression and limited mobility, which lead to soreness and injury. The idea that your legs can work separately, with no pressing or clamping, allows the upper body to move freely and rebalance itself. The lower half of your body drapes over the horse instead of gripping to stay on.

To Work the Legs: The Ta-Daa Technique

To achieve this, Peggy has developed the Ta-Daa Technique. Ta-Daa (as in, "one-two") is an alternating vibration of your legs on the ribs of the horse, which encourages softening of the spine. This in turn induces movement and allows the horse to soften its frame, move forward and lighten to the leg. Peggy developed this technique to replace the squeeze or press on the horse's barrel.

"Ta-Daa" is first best experienced on the trampoline. To learn and better understand the technique, gently bounce on a trampoline if you have one (an exercise mini-tramp is what we have in mind). This imitates the horse's motion and your ability to follow. You begin alternating your legs slightly as if walking in place with soles remaining on the trampoline; follow the bounce with slightly bent knees. Once you get the rhythm, you can relax with the movement. Releasing your back while you are bouncing increases the freedom. Compare bouncing with a tight back or stiff knees and note the difference in the bounce and following the movement.

This exercise leads to the "Ta-Daa" technique mounted. "Ta-Daa" is a brief alternating shiver in the leg motion that sends the horse forward with little effort from the rider. Once it is learned the technique goes undetected by the observer.

However, if a horse is really "stuck" in its body, you may have to intensify the movement. Once the horse moves, you can go back to the gentle pulsations and more subtle leg aids.

3. Allow the Neck and Back to Soften

With the instructor or a friend holding your ankle and bringing your leg slightly back and under you, take a deep breath and let it out. The rider should concentrate on allowing her neck and back to relax. The person on the ground should let your leg slowly drop as she feels a change. Subsequently, the leg will "melt" and begin to drop on its own into a relaxed position. The assistant will feel your leg lengthen and drop into balance.

4. Spring in the Hinges

Have your instructor place a hand under your foot just behind the ball. Relax and allow the assistant to bounce your

The rider should concentrate on allowing her neck and back to relax while the instructor holds her leg. Once the relaxing begins, the leg will also relax and lengthen.

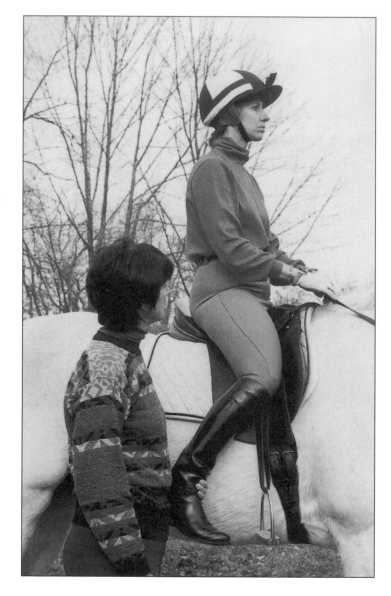

leg up and down and around. The hinges are working and there is a spring to all of the joints.

While your leg is being bounced from the area behind the ball of the foot, it should feel light and springy. The rider experiences the movement of the horse from her leg being bounced as if her foot were in the stirrup and she were trotting or cantering.

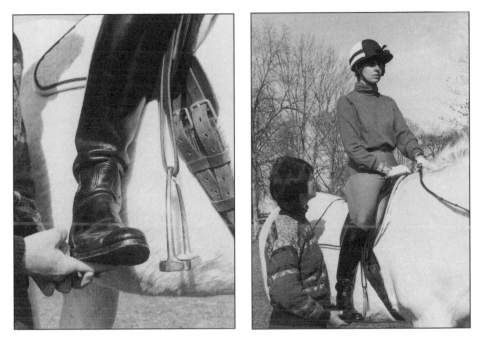

In order for the rider to understand how her hinges work with motion, Peggy holds her finger, as if it were the stirrup, behind the ball of the foot and bounces the leg of the rider.

5. Balanced Feet

Imagine a continuous, even water flow from your head to your toes. If there are any closed joints, they act like kinks in a hose; the water flow stops, and the areas below become dehydrated and stop moving. The ankle remains flexible when the foot is parallel to the ground, and the ball joint behind the toes is able to flex. The stirrup should be just behind the ball joint so you maintain flexibility and movement.

6. Stretchy Elbows

This movement teaches you how to meet the horse and change its unwanted behavior whether it is pulling, dropping the bit or being inconsistent.

In this exercise, horse and rider and a handler practice together. The rider establishes a light contact in a balanced position with elbows bent. The handler imitates the horse and applies pressure to the reins or slackens them, as the horse would. Once the rider meets the contact equally,

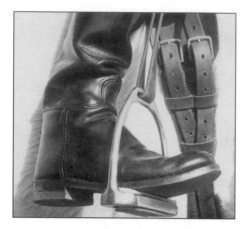

A well-balanced foot, front view.

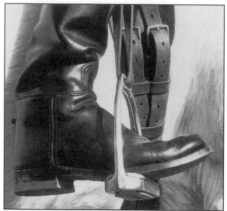

A well-balanced foot, side view.

she very slowly softens the contraction of the arm muscles. (Count from ten backwards, using the count as a slow release.) The rider slowly slides her elbows backward toward the sides of her body and maintains the contact.

As you apply this exercise in motion, it becomes more valuable because it teaches you to maintain the contact by meeting and slowly softening. Meet and melt within the motion of the horse's head. Once again this brings the partnership back into balance.

Peggy Cummings acts as the horse would by pulling on the reins. She instructs the rider to meet the mouth by stretching the elbow backward to equal the pressure and then slowly melt by softening the muscles under the arms and rib cage.

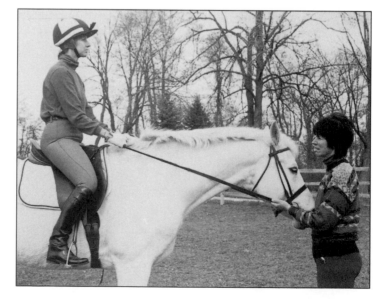

7. Arms and Shoulders Awareness

Bring both hands down to your side and let your arms dangle. Now turn your *palms up* and notice how your arms move while hanging down. Turn the palms out and under, and repeat a couple of times to develop body awareness. Notice the rotation of the hand melts the tense shoulder. There is no clamping in the armpit after this exercise.

Another helpful exercise works through imaging. Imagine you are inside a fish tank, and touch the walls parallel to your ears. Push against the wall, hold for a few seconds, relax and repeat. This exercise softens the collar bone and shoulder area. Slowly bring your arms back around into the riding position. You will find they lie flat against your body, and your joints remain more flexible.

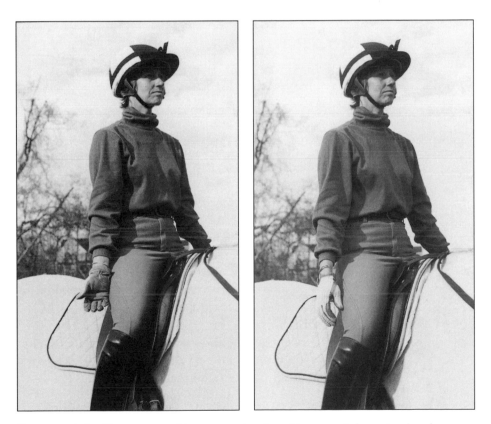

For arm and shoulder awareness, let your arms dangle and turn your palms out and under. Repeat. Notice how your shoulder relaxes with the slow rotation.

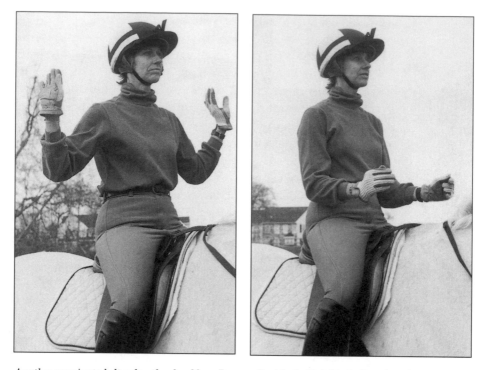

Another exercise to help relax the shoulders. Peggy calls this the Fish Tank. Imagine placing your palms high against the walls of a fish tank and sliding down slowly to shoulder height. Repeat. Slowly bring arms back around to riding position.

8. Open the Shoulders

One of Peggy's best exercises for the shoulders uses a bubble gum image. Picture a piece of soft bubble gum sitting on top of each shoulder. Now place your fingers on the gum and pull it slowly up and out with bent elbows, and imagine that string of bubble gum following. Then slowly bring your arms down the sides of your body and around until your elbows are resting at your sides and your hands are in the correct position over the withers. This puts you in a relaxed position with shoulders centered and square over your hips.

At the beginning of the exercise, the arms feel heavy, but when you breathe and let the arms down slowly, they will automatically lighten and feel more open.

9. Rebalance by "Floating"

To further achieve balance and the ability to regain balance, use the image of "floating" forward with your chest. Take in a deep breath and imagine blowing out a candle positioned between the horse's ears, slowly allowing your chest to soften and feeling your back fill as you exhale. It's actually releasing through the back and hip and brings your whole body into balance.

Looking at horse and rider from the side, picture the face of a clock and a line running from 12 through 6. This line would indicate perfect balance, a center line or a plumb line. Think about the side view of a rider, with a plumb line drawn from her ear, through the shoulder, hip and ankle. This is a centered or ideal balanced position at 12 noon.

If you are one to two minutes before 12, you are behind the motion and need to "float" your body to regain the balanced position. This exercise and imagery will assist you in your rebalancing efforts at any speed.

I remember watching Peggy give a lesson to an Advanced Level three-day event rider who was working on improving her dressage scores. "Floating" seemed to be the one exercise that made all of the difference in her otherwise rough transitions. The rider commented later that she reminds herself to "float" all the time now and it has made a tremendous difference in her performance. This one tiny tool can make a major impact for any rider.

Translate the Traditional

As a fellow rider, I don't expect you to forget everything you've learned and start over. But I do hope you will at least begin thinking about a balanced position by incorporating some of these techniques and exercises into your traditional program. What this is all about is combining a new understanding of women's physical capabilities and needs with a new set of techniques designed to enhance performance and enjoyment. That means taking what works for you and adding it to your program. Ideally, you'll see results that lead you to incorporate more and more as your riding (and pleasure from it) improves.

If you are wondering how all of this can work for you in a traditional setting, it is possible. Learning to ride in balance and with motion should be the basis of all riding. Once the basics are in place, "layers" can be added as you progress in your discipline. You will always be one step ahead in your training and more comfortable doing so.

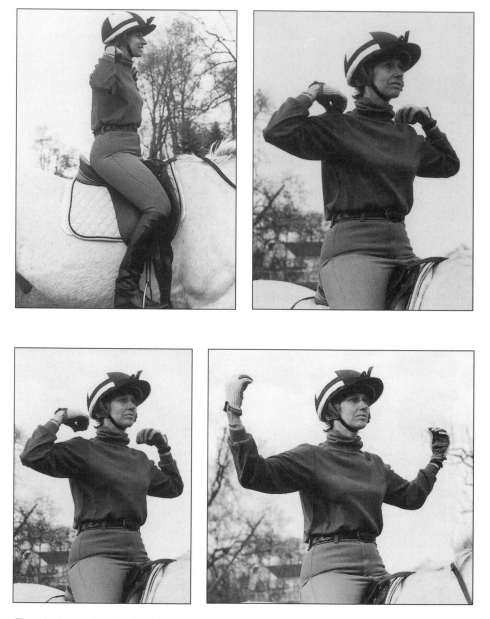

To assist in opening the shoulder and collar bone structures, try Peggy's Bubble Gum Shoulder Exercise. The rider imagines a wad of bubble gum on the top of each shoulder. By picking up the gum with each hand simultaneously, the rider slowly lifts the string of gum (it's still stuck to your shoulders) up, out, around and down until her hands are in the riding position.

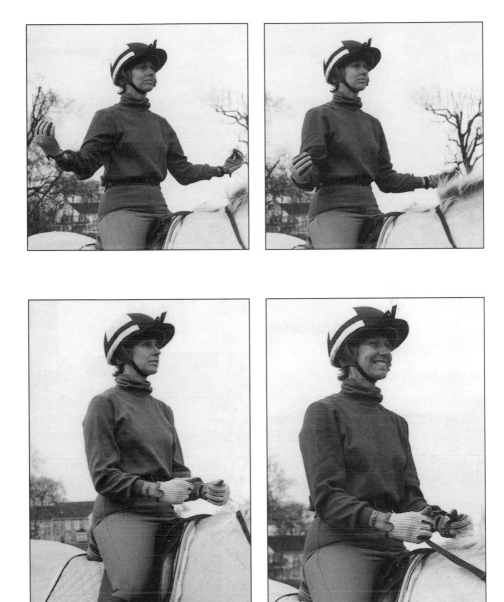

Peggy has set up a number of instructor clinics to show teachers how to work with their students and "translate" traditional commands into images and language their students can understand. She also works with students so that they can "translate" what their instructor at home is asking for and do what works for themselves and their bodies. Here are a few examples to show you how you can achieve performance through the translation of traditional commands.

Traditional Command	Peggy's In-Balance Riding
"Sit up"	Breathe and float; let chest soften.
"Half halt"	Float, release the back, stretch elbow, and meet and melt with the contact. (Varying degrees of these techniques are necessary depending on the horse.)
"More leg"	When clamping or pressing with the lower leg, the upper leg is lost and the lower back tightens. Float and release, which allows the upper leg to move and the lower leg to be free to give the pulsating rhythm that encourages impulsion. Use the Ta-Daa Technique. It feels like you are helping a ball bounce between the legs.
"Check and Give"	Meet and melt with the contact.

As you begin to incorporate these exercises and input "new" information into your body, a natural imprinting takes place. It's as if your body is thanking you for reverting back to your natural relaxed, flexible state: "Oh yeah, that's how it's supposed to work." You have to work at undoing what you have been doing for years, but the body knows how it wants to work and will be more responsive. I have been learning and practicing these techniques for a few years now, and they work for me without much mental or physical effort on my part. I still have to play my mental tapes to remind myself to breathe and relax, but it is becoming second nature. I am learning to "allow" my body to work with the horse. It's what the body and the horse want and need to perform as a team.

Riding in or out of balance is something you must experience and learn to feel. We can describe what is happening and show you pictures, but you have to feel it to learn it. Only you can know when your body is in harmony with your horse.

We have gotten too far away from what comes naturally in riding, and finding it again is a relief! We are born with innate release, resiliency and balancing abilities, but seem to lose them progressively along life's path. The tension, soreness, pain and frustration that result from this loss need not be a part of riding, provided we make the effort to re-gain and refine these qualities. A female rider with a bal-anced position and a flexible body is able to respond more effectively in lessons, in the show ring, on the trail, working cattle or in any horse-related situation.

Peggy's work is so gratifying to her and to all of us in-volved with her because we have yet to see anything but positive results. When the messages are clear, you maximize performance. In emergencies, you survive because of the communication.

Peggy Cummings' Formula for Success and Fun: Free Horse and Free Rider

Women and horses pay a high price for a lack of knowledge. The good news is that with AWAREness, we can *release* our old habits and the rigidity in our bodies, born of teachings that don't work; we can re-connect with our own bodies, with our horses and with our original vision of what the horse/human relationship should be; we can move out of the force/fear/pain/resistance/force cycle, into freedom. And from that place, we can each allow the dance to begin.

"Free Horse" Equation

Balance + Freedom of Motion under Saddle = Self-Carriage	
Rider Goal	An aid, not an encumbrance
Horse Goal	A "following" dance partner
Keys to Success	Balanced shoeing
	Level and properly fitted saddle
	Correct tack fit and usage
	Health, nutrition, teeth, conditioning and environment
	Size and temperament

"Free Rider"

Clear Interaction and Communication with Horse = Balance and Freedom of Motion in Body

Rider Goal	A "leading" dance partner
Horse Goal	Self-carriage
Keys to Success	Dynamic* alignment of ear, shoulder, hip and ankle in a balanced seat
	"Released" hinges and spine, soft lower back
	Ability to continually regain balance in motion
	Regularity of rhythm for horse and support system for rebalancing
	Facilitate freedom of motion rather than inhibiting it
	Health, nutrition, fitness and flexibility
	(*in rhythm and motion)

Chapter 5

Common Injuries and
Their Causes

*I believe that to be perfectly cool on all occasions, never to be flurried,
or taken unaware, and above all things never to lose temper, no
matter how trying the circumstances, will best ensure successful
equestrianism, both for men and women. To expect to ride without
encountering difficulties and worries, as well as risks and dangers,
is only to look for something that cannot possibly be attained.*
—Mrs. Power O'Donoghue, *Riding for Ladies*, 1887

*A*ll athletes encounter injury at some point, but the best
of them anticipate the challenge and do everything they
can to avoid injury. Generally, that means taking care of
yourself and preparing your body for the work to be done.
Prevention is the key, and my approach here is to identify
what can go wrong and, later, to suggest what to do to prevent it in the first place.

You are an equestrian athlete. You too have to meet the
challenge of physical problems if you want to get the most
out of riding. If we understand how most injuries occur, we
can prepare ourselves with specific equipment, clothing,
flexibility movements and strengthening exercises, decreasing the chance that we'll suffer pain and have to spend
time away from our horses. Prevention starts with appropriate training both when mounted and on the ground,
choosing the right horse and utilizing and maintaining your
equipment properly, all of which serve to decrease the
incidence of avoidable soreness and disability.

Falls and barn hazards account for the high-visibility injuries; they will be addressed later in this book. For now, let's examine a less recognized but nonetheless substantial volume of injuries that occurs simply from the rigors of riding and the wear and tear of caring for your horse. Here again, awareness of your body and its limitations is the first line of defense, followed closely by the ability to recognize the early signs of injury.

Buddies lifting together minimizes body strain.

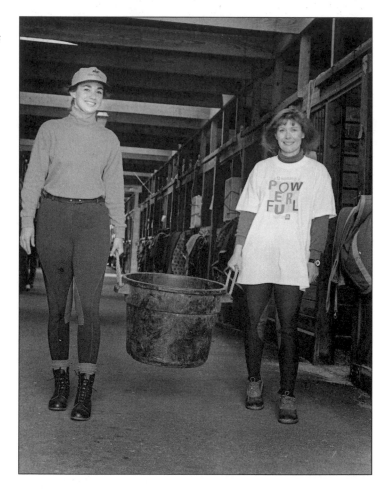

Common Injuries

While the purpose of what follows is to address causes, remember that persistent pain warrants a trip to your physician or physical therapist to get an assessment of your condition.

Low back pain is the most common complaint of female riders. The cause is twofold: poor body mechanics—for example, doing barn and house chores without using your legs and bending your knees—and poor flexibility throughout the lower body and trunk, which creates a stiff, nonshock-absorbing seat. The most common disorders in younger riders are compression fractures and injuries to the intervertebral discs. Spinal stenosis and the effects of arthritis are more common in mature women.

Disc injuries occur with repetitive forward bending, a slouched posture, poor hip flexibility and poor control of trunk muscles. What occurs with repeated forward bending and inflexibility is continued backward motion on the posterior of the disc. Recall our analogy to the jelly donut: If you compress one side of the donut, the jelly will bulge out the other side; do it repeatedly, and you've got a mess. The same phenomenon essentially takes place when a "slipped disc" occurs. The disc bulges in the back, creating pressure on the nerve, which in turn culminates in a variety of painful symptoms in the back and down the leg. Disc injury can easily be avoided by maintaining good spinal alignment (good posture) and following these basic rules:

- Learn to maintain proper spinal alignment.

- Support your spine by contracting your abdominal muscles while lifting.

- Keep the object close to you as you lift.

- Keep a wide base of support for balance as you squat down to lift (widen your base of support by extending a "support hand" when you have to reach for something).

- Shift your weight as you push or pull.

- Shift your weight up and down when you lift.

Compression fractures typically result from a fall or extreme concussion. They create a wedge-type deformity within the vertebrae, limiting some of the natural motion. These fractures are painful and will keep you from riding for approximately two months, but they do not usually cause any nerve damage or other permanent damage.

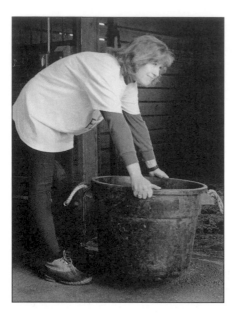

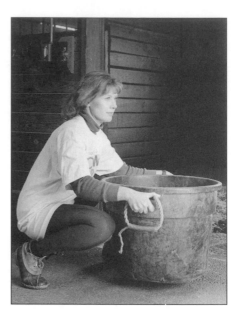

Leslie Wood demonstrates the incorrect and potentially dangerous way to pick up an object.

Correct and comfortable way to pick up a basket.

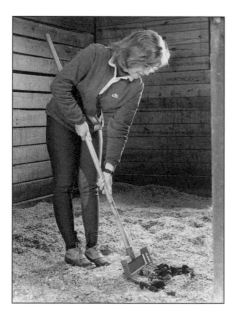

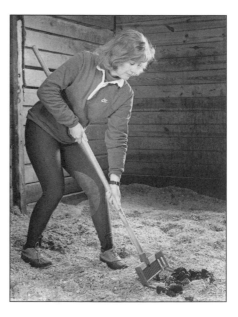

Mucking out the wrong way.

Mucking out using your "hinges" correctly.

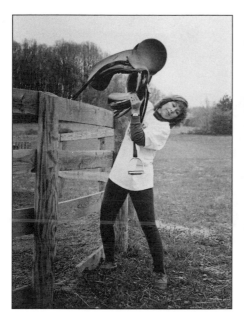 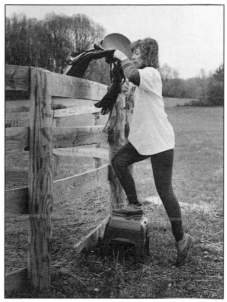

Lifting a heavy object overhead incorrectly. *Leslie uses a stool this time—what a relief!*

Rehabilitation includes flexibility and postural strengthening exercises, with emphasis on supporting the spine.

Arthritis is essentially a result of wear and tear on a joint. The symptoms can include pain with range of motion and compression on the spine. Rehabilitation includes range-of-motion, flexibility and strengthening exercises designed to help to support the joint. Many riders find that a low-back support is useful at times to keep the area warm and therefore more supple and provides an added degree of stability while good muscular support is established.

Spinal stenosis is the calcification and narrowing of the canal through which the nerves of the spinal cord and the nerve roots pass. This is a naturally occurring phenomenon, but certain vertebrae may be more involved if there is a history of trauma to that area, for example, a fall or a previous disc problem. Spinal stenosis occurs as we age, thus the focus on an active lifestyle is important for maintaining normal flexibility and strength to minimize the effects of this aging process.

AWAREness

Back supports can help in healing and strengthening, but they don't take the place of an exercise program.

Rider holding her head forward, which begins a vicious cycle that leads to an out-of-balance rider in a great deal of pain.

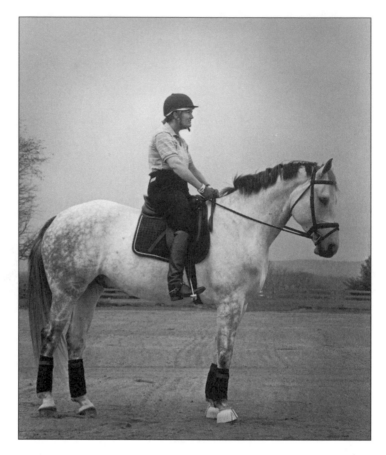

Neck and upper back pain is a very common problem in female riders. The primary cause is slouching, which promotes a forward head posture and rounded shoulders.

Note the rider's head position in a forward posture. This position incorrectly places the head (which weighs about 15 pounds in the average woman!) out of good spinal alignment, and a vicious cycle begins. This head position puts undue pressure on the intervertebral discs at the base of the neck, very much like what constant forward bending does to the lower back. It also creates a biomechanical disadvantage for the muscles that support the spine at the base of the neck, making these muscles work extra hard to keep the head up. If you took gymnastics as a child, you may remember the teacher telling you

---

AWAREness

Your head can throw everything in the chain out of sync. Not only do you have to use your head when you're riding; you have to position it properly as well.

---

that your body will follow your head. The forward head posture also leads to the forward rounded shoulder position. This position creates strain in the upper back and inhibits the natural movement of the shoulder girdle, preventing the movement that must occur for your hands to be most effective. (Recall also our discussion of back release in the previous chapter.)

Typically this posture leads to what I refer to as "monkey riders." Their shoulders are forward and they ride with their elbows out, breaking the normal line that should run from the reins through the hand up to the elbow. Technically, in riding the motions of the hand aid emanate from the forward and backward motion of the shoulder, thus maintaining the proper alignment that is essential to effective aids and balanced riding.

Essentially, all the ailments that affect the lumbar spine also affect the cervical spine, which is the neck. Prevention simply involves good posture and strengthening the upper back muscles through exercise.

Shoulder injuries, specifically rotator cuff injuries, are also common in women. The rotator cuff muscles are the muscles that help to support the shoulder and sustain good biomechanics. As you raise your hand over your head, the rotator cuff rotates the humerus to prevent interference with the joint. Rotator cuff injuries often occur with repetitive activity at shoulder height or above, such as lifting or repetitive work such as grooming.

AWAREness

Accidents account for a smaller percentage of injuries than you may think.

Women typically do not have adequate strength in the upper body, but as horsewomen we still perform all the heavy chores required for the upkeep of a horse and barn. This combination, along with the cumulative trauma and the effects of age, leaves female equestrians particularly susceptible to this kind of injury.

Hip and knee problems are not usually a direct result of riding. In many cases, however, a rider may have a predisposition to knee pain based on a pre-existing condition. The position and movement of riding might exacerbate the problem. As mentioned earlier, anterior knee pain is very common in women due to the increased angle of the hip to the knee. With a poorly aligned knee, sitting on a horse with the knee flexed for long periods, or continually bending and straightening the knee (as in the rising trot), can cause increased rubbing of the kneecap, resulting in pain and stiffness.

A way to prevent this is to perform exercises that strengthen the inner muscles of the knee. Also, to alleviate some of the stiffness, take your feet out of the stirrups and move your legs around frequently to maintain their flexibility.

Hip pain primarily occurs with insufficient flexibility and poor saddle fit. The saddle should be evaluated for the correct fit to ensure comfort for the horse and rider. The size of the horse also plays a role. If you are a petite woman and have a very wide-barreled horse, you may feel there is more strain on your hips when you position your leg.

Pubic area (genital or soft tissue) injuries affect most women riders at one time or another, but they are often too shy or intimidated to discuss them. Most women have at one time or another suffered from saddle sores, for example. When a great deal of friction occurs, the soft tissue of the pubic area may even swell to the point of discouraging urination. The causes are typically poor biomechanics of the seat, which create friction and constant rubbing, especially at the fork of the seat; improper saddle fit; riding for a longer period of time than you are used to; and riding at the sitting trot for an extended period of time.

Biomechanically, the friction is caused by a stiff, immobile hip and lower back and the rider not "going with the movement of the horse," or overriding the movement of the horse. The first thing to keep in mind is that it will get better as you work through the problem and adjust your equipment. Powders are very useful in absorbing perspiration and can decrease friction in this area. Powders with baking soda are especially recommended.

Lingerie and underwear specially designed for the woman rider can greatly reduce friction and chafing. (For more on this, see chapter 7.)

Not surprisingly, the saddle is the primary source of discomfort. But it's not the saddle's fault. Proper saddle fit, extensively discussed in chapter 7, is vital to healthy and happy riding. Saddles that incorporate female body dynamics in their design elements are now available.

Breast injury is a logical consequence of inadequate support. A support bra is essential for all female athletes, including riders, regardless of breast size. Riding is a high-impact sport with a significant amount of bounce. The breasts are supported by a series of ligaments. Once these ligaments become overstretched, they do not return to their original shape. This most commonly affects women as they age, but does not exclude younger riders. All females, from puberty through adult life, should wear support undergarments for high impact sports such as riding.

If you pay attention to the early warning signs of any of the problems described above, you'll be well on the way to dealing with them with minimal pain, frustration and lost riding time. For more serious injury or trauma, it is very important that you locate a health-care professional who is familiar with the rigors of riding in order to create the best rehabilitation program.

More specifically, the issues we've been talking about boil down to proper technique and equipment, including clothing. Now that we've detailed most of the unpleasantness, we can get on with the business of describing how best to prepare for the riding experience.

Generally speaking, physical problems have a common solution: prevention.

Chapter 6

Exercises for Your Half of the Partnership

For women, quite as much as and even more than for men, it [riding] is of all exercises the one best adapted to keep them in condition, to restore the glow of health, and to key up the whole system to respond to all the delights of life.—Belle Beach, *Riding and Driving for Women*, 1912

If you want to be successful with horses, you have to make a physical commitment. That means putting some extra effort into preparing for the demands of riding.

I have found that no other single activity is as beneficial to women as riding for overall physical fitness and muscle development. Riding promotes good posture and naturally strengthens your abdominal, back and thigh muscles. If you take any time off from regular riding, you notice the change immediately. No matter how much I jog or work out with weights or toning machines, I can't seem to get the same positive shaping results I do with riding. Riding strengthens and trims simultaneously. And riding has the added bonus of providing mental therapy.

Just because we're sitting when we ride does not mean we are not active. Riding is an extremely athletic activity. People who don't think it is typically haven't gotten anywhere near a horse, and certainly not on top of one with the intent of propelling it forward. The degree to which it works for you depends on how much you put into it—as with any sport or other physical effort.

Part of what we love about riding and being around horses is the opportunity to get outside in the fresh air, to get physical, to feel fit. Riding requires both physical ability in the saddle and hard work in preparation for those minutes in the saddle. For most of us, the combination works well.

Everyone who rides, however, should incorporate a cross-training program and proper nutrition in their regimen to stay fit and healthy and prevent injury.

We know that men have more muscle mass in their upper body than women. We tend to be lighter through our upper bodies and have to work hard to maintain upper-body strength. We also have the tendency to overuse our upper bodies without building a support system, leading to the variety of pains and inflammations described in the last chapter. By carrying full water buckets, moving hay bales and feed bags, lifting heavy saddles high above our heads and grooming 17-hand horses, women are likely to experience pain and accumulate nagging injuries. If done improperly, without the tools available to assist us, chores can prevent us from riding at our best. Improper riding technique, coupled with a lack of physical preparation, will do the same.

Equestrians seem less likely than other athletes to stretch prior to exertion and to use exercise to enhance performance. The following stretching and strengthening program was designed for a woman's special needs as an equestrian.

Stretching

Stretching is the one form of exercise that many athletes don't understand, forget to do or simply don't know how to perform properly. And it is the most essential.

AWAREness

Stretching simultaneously brings energy and relaxation to your body.

The purpose of stretching is to prepare the muscles and joints for the activity they are about to perform. A good stretch requires the intended muscle to be isolated without compromising any of the surrounding joints. This means maintaining good form throughout the stretch. To achieve the desired effect, the stretch must reach the comfortable "end range" of the muscle without inducing pain. It is up to you to identify where your thresholds are to maximize the stretch without causing damage; build those thresholds progressively, a little at a time, to increase the flexibility and strength of the muscle.

Remember:

- The stretch should be maintained for at least ten seconds.

- No "bouncing" or ballistic-type movements.

- Each stretch should be repeated at least once.

- Stretching should be performed daily, even if you don't plan to ride.

Here are some pre- and post-riding stretches. Mary Beth Walsh, our physical therapist, recommends that all riders perform this short, comprehensive group of stretches regardless of age or riding discipline.

The Quad Stretch demonstrated by Gwyn Donohue. Grab your ankle with your knee bent, and gently pull your knee back. Make sure you don't allow your back to arch.

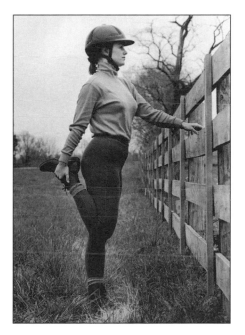

1. Front of the Thigh (Quadriceps) Stretch

The quadriceps muscle is in the front of the thigh. It is necessary for this muscle to be flexible to allow the leg to fall easily under the pelvis and allow movement of the hip joint. It is especially helpful for activities that require a "long leg," such as dressage, western pleasure and endurance riding.

Grab your ankle with your knee bent, and gently pull your knee back. Make sure you don't allow your back to arch. Hold ten seconds. Pause and repeat.

2. Front of Hip to Thigh (Iliopsoas) Stretch

The iliopsoas muscle is in the front of the hip and connects to the upper portion of the thigh. This is a very tight area for most women and this stretch can have a tremendous benefit on your flexibility in the saddle.

In the half-kneeling position, lean or lunge forward to feel the stretch in the front of the hip. Keep your feet pointed forward and hold ten seconds. Pause and repeat.

Iliopsoas Muscle Stretch. Lean or lunge forward onto one leg with feet facing forward. This will stretch the muscle between the hip and the front of the thigh.

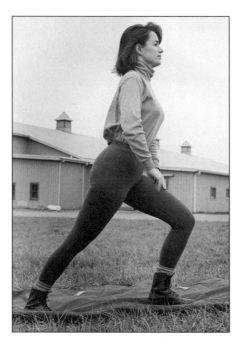

3. Back of Thigh (Hamstring) Stretch

The hamstring muscles are in the back part of the thigh. If these muscles are tight, they cause the lower back to flatten and restrict motion, creating a concussive position.

A. Seated, extend one leg straight in front of you; keeping the back straight, bend forward over that leg. Do not

Seated Hamstring Stretch. Seated, extend one leg straight in front of you; keeping the back straight, bend forward over that leg. Do not round your back; keep it flat and look ahead.

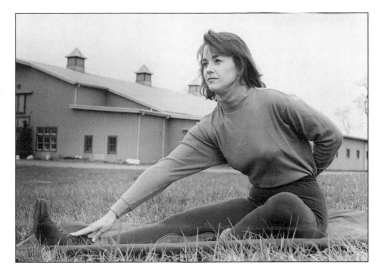

round your back; keep it flat and look ahead. Hold ten seconds. Pause and repeat.

or

B. Standing, place one foot on a stool or fence in front of you; keeping your back straight, bend forward over the leg. Hold ten seconds. Pause and repeat.

Standing Hamstring Stretch. Standing, place one foot on a stool or fence in front of you. Keeping the back straight, bend forward over the leg.

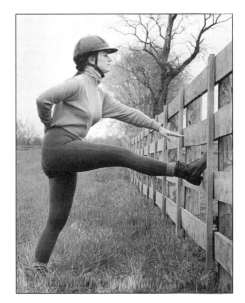

or

C. Lying down on your back, lift one leg straight up with a slightly bent knee, hold the leg behind the knee with both hands and gently pull the leg toward you. Hold ten seconds. Pause and repeat. This stretch is very effective for every kind of riding.

Lying-down Hamstring Stretch. Lying down on your back, lift one leg straight up with a slightly bent knee. Hold the leg behind the knee with both hands and gently pull the leg toward you.

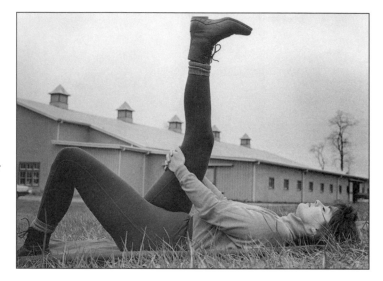

4. Inner Thigh (Adductor) Stretch

The adductor muscles are the muscles of the inner thigh. If these muscles are tight, they prevent the rider from achieving a deep and relaxed seat.

Inner Thigh Stretch. Seated, bring the soles of your feet together. Take a deep breath and spend a few seconds allowing the hip joint to relax. Gently press down on one or both knees until you feel a stretch.

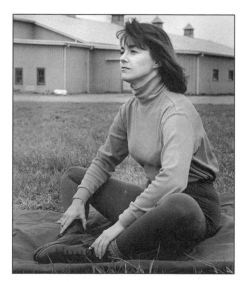

Seated, bring the soles of the feet together, take a deep breath and spend a few seconds to let the hip joint relax. Gently press down on one or both knees until you feel a stretch. Hold ten seconds. Pause and repeat.

Stretch for the Inner Thigh. Lie on your back with both knees up. Bring one leg up and place your ankle on the other knee. Now gently press on the knee that is up, to stretch the muscles in the inner thigh.

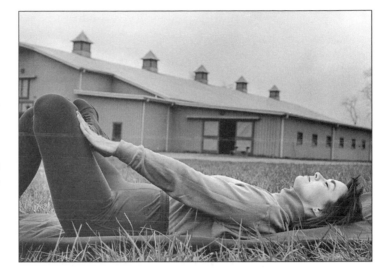

5. Buttock (Piriformis) Stretch

This addresses a deep buttock muscle that causes the leg to turn out. If this muscle is tight, it will be difficult to allow the leg to fall into the correct position.

Lying down on your back with one leg bent, pull the bent knee across the body toward the opposite shoulder until you feel a stretch in the buttock. Hold ten seconds. Pause and repeat.

Piriformis Stretch. Lying down on your back with one leg bent, pull the bent knee across the body toward the opposite shoulder until you feel a stretch in the buttock.

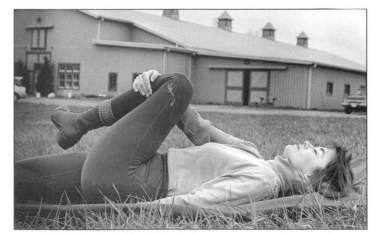

6. Calf (Gastrocnemius and Soleus) Stretch

These are the muscles of the calf. If these muscles are tight, they prevent the heel from relaxing.

Stand with one foot in front of the other as in a lunge position. Keep the heel of the back leg down and gently stretch forward. Hold ten seconds. Pause and repeat.

Calf Stretch. Stand with one foot in front of the other, as in a lunge position. Keep the heel of the back leg down and gently stretch forward.

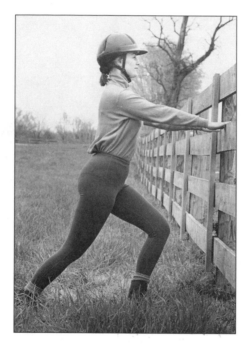

7. Lower Back Stretch

There are three different types of stretches for the lower back. The first stretches the paravertebral muscles that lie on either side of the backbone. The second and third help reduce pressure on the disc and help restore the lordosis of the lower spine.

Note that all three of these exercises should be performed in sets of ten rather than holding the position for ten seconds. Also, the standing backward bend is useful to perform periodically to relieve strain on the back while performing barn chores.

A. Lying down, bring both legs up to your abdomen and gently pull your knees closer to you. Perform ten repetitions.

Lower Back Stretch. Lying down, bring both legs up to your abdomen and gently pull your knees closer to you.

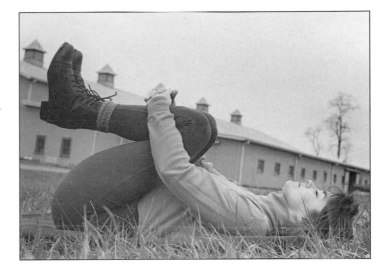

B. Lying on your stomach, place your hands as if you were going to do a pushup. Press up with your upper body but keep your hips on the ground. Perform ten repetitions.

Lower Back Stretch. Lying on your stomach, place your hands as if you were going to perform a pushup. Press up with your upper body, but keep your hips on the ground.

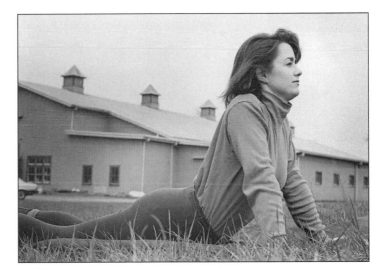

C. Standing, place your hands in the small of your back and arch backward. Perform ten repetitions.

Lower Back Stretch. Standing, place your hands in the small of your back and arch backward.

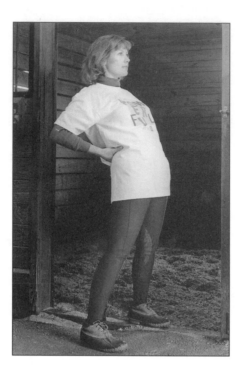

8. Mid-Trunk Stretch

The mid-trunk or thoracic spine is chiefly responsible for the rotation of the back. This motion is necessary to perform lateral work correctly.

Seated, with weight evenly distributed on both seat bones, place one hand behind the back, the other on the opposite shoulder. Gently rotate the trunk and stretch. Switch hands and work on the other side. For an additional stretch, place one hand behind the head and arch backwards against a chair until you feel a stretch.

9. Neck Stretch

The best stretch for the neck is to perform a Chin Tuck to stretch the cervical paravertebral muscles. This allows you to keep your head over your shoulders in proper position.

Place your fingertips on your chin and gently push your chin back like a drawer until you feel a gentle stretch in the back of the neck. Hold for ten seconds and repeat up to ten times.

Chin Tuck. Place your fingertips on your chin and gently push your chin back like a drawer until you feel a gentle stretch in the back of the neck.

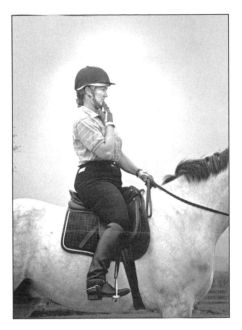

10. Side (Latissimus Dorsi and Triceps) Stretch
These are the muscles of the shoulder and lateral back. If these muscles are tight, they restrict rotation and movement of the shoulder.

Side Stretch. Standing, raise one arm up and over the head, and lean over to one side.

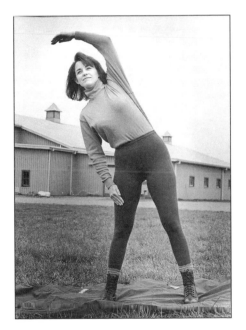

Standing, raise one arm up over the head and lean over to one side. Hold ten seconds. Pause and repeat. To include the triceps muscle of the arm, grab one elbow with your opposite hand and pull it over and behind the head.

To include the triceps muscle of the arm, grab one elbow and pull it over the head with the side stretch.

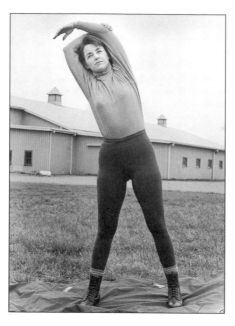

Leslie Wood demonstrates the Pectoral Stretch. Stand in a doorway with the arms stretched overhead or at shoulder height. Slowly lean forward and hold.

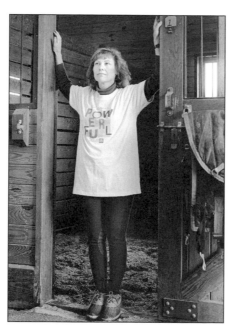

11. Chest (Pectoral) Muscle Stretch

These are the muscles of the chest, which if restricted prevent the shoulders from being positioned in proper alignment. Note: You should not perform this stretch if you have ever sustained a dislocation injury to the shoulder.

Stand in a doorway with the arms stretched overhead or at shoulder height. Slowly lean forward.

Strengthening Exercises

A strengthening program is needed to keep fit during the off-season as well as to maintain strength in primary and support muscles, whether you ride occasionally or full-time. Think about exercising as a get-fit-to-ride activity.

Anyone who tries a new sport can attest to the fact that you use more muscles and expend more energy while you are learning the game. Once the appropriate muscles are developed, things get easier. Nonetheless, any participant needs to supplement the activity with an exercise program to maximize results. That's because the additional support muscles can be developed to improve performance and endurance.

Besides nerves, novice riders expend more energy and effort trying to figure out what muscles to use and how to do multiple tasks at once. People often ask, "What type of strength does riding improve?" and "Is riding an aerobic activity?" The answer is that it depends on the level, intensity and activity. Going around a ring for thirty minutes is insufficient as a cardiovascular workout, but any endurance rider will tell you that riding a course certainly gets her heart rate going.

You will need to regulate the amount and intensity of exercise in accordance with your riding time, level and requirements. You should first be aware that unless you ride regularly (four to five times per week) and achieve a *target heart rate* (see chart) for at least thirty minutes per ride, you are not receiving any real cardiovascular training. You need to supplement your riding with a cross-training activity or exercise program to ensure your own fitness level.

You prepare and maintain your horse for work and performance; you should do the same for *yourself*. It's a 50-50 deal!

Cross-training is especially useful in preventing exercise burnout and for strengthening a variety of muscle groups. Some cross-training suggestions for riders are swimming, running, cross-country skiing machines (or the real thing) and general aerobics. To get the *maximum* cardiovascular benefit, you should perform an aerobic workout at least three times a week (optimally, five times a week), maintaining a training heart rate for at least twenty minutes.

Realistically, though, any level of workout is better than none. Depending on your schedule, a couple of days of exercise or cross-training activity coupled with two days of riding a week will get you into good shape. If the regimen gets boring or you are feeling fatigued on a regular basis, move on to something different or just give yourself a break for a while. This isn't meant to be punishment. It's up to you to determine your own personal goals and, along with that, how hard to push.

The key is to *build* toward your goal.

Your Maximum Training Heart Rate

Take your heart rate by counting how many beats are in a ten-second period immediately after you exercise. Find a pulse point on your neck or wrist and count your beats per ten seconds. Multiply this times six to find your beats-per-minute heart rate.

Formula	Sample
Base of 220 – your age × 65%	220–40 (years of age) = 180
	180 × .65 = 117
	Initial Target: 117 beats per minute

As you increase your workout to three to five times per week over several weeks, increase the percentage. Move up on your own as you feel comfortable.

For example:

Weeks 1–3	65% = 117
Weeks 3–6	70–75% = 135
Weeks 6 and on	85% = 153 MAX

The maximum training heart rate is 85 percent. Do not go above 85 percent.

Heart Rate Target Workout Rates

	Target Rates						
Age	**65%**	**75%**	**85%**	**Age**	**65%**	**75%**	**85%**
18	131	152	172	44	114	132	150
20	130	150	170	46	113	131	148
22	129	149	168	48	112	129	146
24	127	147	167	50	111	128	145
26	126	146	165	52	109	126	143
28	125	144	163	54	108	125	141
30	124	143	162	56	107	123	139
32	122	141	160	58	105	122	138
34	121	140	158	60	104	120	136
36	120	138	156	65	101	116	132
38	118	137	155	70	98	113	128
40	117	135	153	75	94	109	123
42	116	134	151				

You will need to increase these exercises as you increase the level and requirements of your sport. A higher level of training is essential for foxhunting, cross-country and especially endurance and race riding.

There is no substitute for hours in the saddle in developing the "feel" for riding. The exercises that I have included starting on page 95 will help you get where you're going faster, and reduce the risk of injury along the way.

Riding involves both isometric and isotonic muscle strength. Isometric contraction of muscle occurs when we contract a muscle and no movement occurs, such as when we use our inner leg on the horse (if done properly, no real movement of the leg occurs). Conversely, isotonic contractions are performed when we move a body part, such as in the rising trot, when we move our pelvis forward and back.

Some aspects of riding entail both types of muscle contractions at the same time. Jumping uses our seat with an isometric contraction of the muscles of our lower leg while our upper body, moving with the horse over the fence, performs an isotonic contraction. Polo is another good example of stabilizing the seat while the lower body and upper body are dynamically moving. Barrel racing requires an immense amount of isometric strength to keep yourself in the saddle.

Simply riding out on a relaxing trail ride does not require the same amount of strength or energy expenditure as some of the activities just mentioned. Still, every rider should be prepared for a worst-case scenario and be fit enough to handle any situation that might occur.

AWAREness

A few minutes of strengthening exercises will prevent days of rehab time.

Strengthening exercises should be performed a maximum of three times weekly and at least once or twice a week, depending on your schedule. If you're very serious about it, alternate day training for strengthening is important, and so is the recovery day when a muscle rejuvenates itself. The combination of regular work and rest creates a truly stronger muscle.

It is important in training to vary the activity from day to day for many reasons, not the least of which is mental! In your riding, for example, perform an endurance interval one day, then on alternate days work on a lunge lesson, which involves more strengthening. Repetition over time, such as day after day of sitting trot work without a break, is similar in effect to a runner pounding the hard pavement without time off: You're going to get hurt. This is especially true as you get older. Therefore, try to mix a variety of activity into your training.

Many women remark that they are always rushing to do something, whether it's barn chores, grooming or riding. Barn chores and grooming certainly count as exercise, but they do not provide any cardiovascular or specific training effect. Adding an exercise program may seem inconceivable in a working rider's life. However, if you perform the simple stretches listed above before you put your foot in the stirrup, or if you set your alarm a few minutes early to perform a few strengthening exercises, you will be ahead of the game in creating and maintaining fitness. (I do my stretches and exercises on weekday evenings while I'm watching television or on the weekends in the mornings.)

The following exercises are designed specifically to strengthen muscles required for all forms of riding. I've included a set of general exercises and a set targeted for different riding disciplines. Finally, there is a set of quick preride warm-ups drawn from our stretching regimen.

Some of the exercises can be done with a Physioball, a durable, therapeutic ball that can be used to strengthen the muscles that support the trunk.[1] Riders find the Physioball especially useful because the motions of the ball simulate the dynamics of the horse, requiring that you stabilize yourself and co-contract the same muscles. Some exercises refer to a Theraband, a stretchy resistive piece of rubber.[2]

If you choose not to use any of these products in your program, you can still perform most of the exercises on the ground or with an appropriate piece of furniture like an ottoman (only a few actually *require* the ball or band). Just ignore the references to the equipment and plow ahead. Or you can concentrate on the other exercises.

General Exercises

1. Abdominals

The abdominal muscles serve to bend the body forward when the pelvis is fixed in place, as in the Abdominal Crunch exercise. The lower abdominals serve to lift the pelvis up when the upper trunk is stabilized. The lower abdominals are very important to riders, especially in dressage, where they serve to control the pelvic motion and prevent an excessive curve in the lower back, which is so common in many female riders.

Abdominal Crunch: While lying on your back, tighten the abdominal muscles so that your lower back is flat against the floor. Bend your knees at roughly a 90-degree angle and position your feet on an appropriate support (couch,

---

[1] For more information on ordering a Physioball, contact Equestrian Resources at P.O. Box 20069, Alexandria, VA, 22320; telephone (703) 836-6353.

[2] Information on Therabands is also available from Equestrian Resources.

ottoman, Physioball). When you get stronger, you can eliminate the support. Keeping the back flat, support your head and neck with your hands. Lift the trunk off the floor about six to eight inches, then lower down, keeping the lower back flat at all times. Do as many as you can up to ten. Pause and repeat.

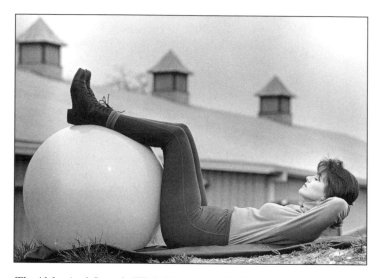

The Abdominal Crunch. While lying on your back, tighten the abdominal muscles so that your lower back is flat against the ground or floor. Keeping the back flat, support your head and neck with your hands. Lift the trunk off the floor about 6 to 8 inches, then lower down, keeping the back flat at all times.

The Reverse Crunch. Lie flat with shoulders down and knees bent. Lift your knees up to your chest. Point your feet, soles upward, and lift the legs and pelvis up toward the ceiling. Imagine pushing the roof up and letting it down.

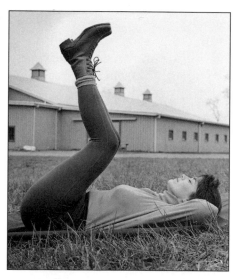

Reverse Crunch: Lie flat with shoulders down and knees bent. Lift your knees up to your chest. Point your feet, soles upward, and lift the legs and pelvis up toward the ceiling, as if pushing the roof up and letting down. Do as many as you can up to ten. Pause and repeat.

Abdominal Obliques: Same exercise as the abdominal crunch, except that when you lift your upper body, move your elbow toward the opposite knee. Do as many as you can up to ten. Pause and repeat.

Abdominal Oblique Strengthening. Use Crunch exercise and rotate toward opposite knee with each lift of the upper body.

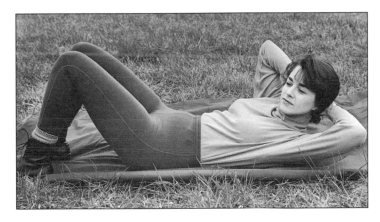

2. Back

Superwoman: This exercise strengthens all the back muscles. Start in a crouched or froglike position, then

The Superwoman. Start in a crouched or frog-like position, then stretch your arms straight out as you lie on the ball.

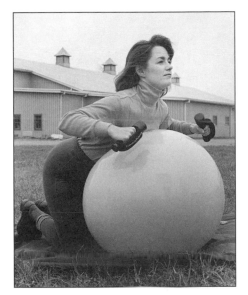

Hold the Superwoman position for five seconds, then resume the crouch position. Add hand weights as needed.

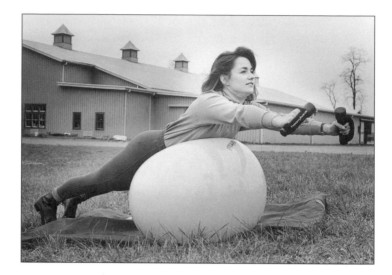

stretch your arms and legs straight out as you lie on the ball. Hold the position for five seconds, then resume the crouch position again. Add hand weights as needed. Repeat in sets of ten.

Prone Flies: Raise elbows up to shoulder height and keep them bent at a 90-degree angle. Raise elbows up and down by squeezing shoulder blades together as you lift. Do as many as you can up to ten. Pause and repeat. Add hand weights as needed.

Prone Fly. Raise elbows up to shoulder height and keep them bent at 90 degrees.

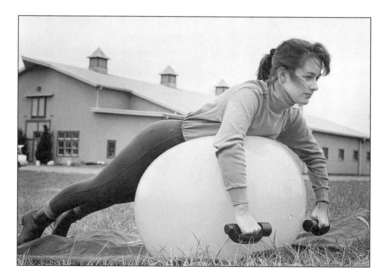

Raise elbows up and down by squeezing shoulder blades together as you lift to complete Prone Flies. Add hand weights as needed.

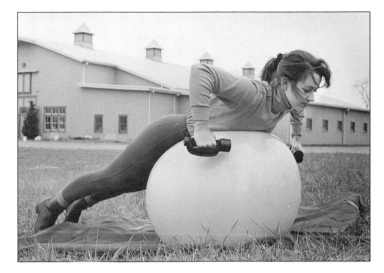

Pushups: On the ball, start on all fours with the ball under your chest and "walk over" it until the ball is under your knees. Perform a typical pushup, taking care to keep the back still. Do as many as you can up to ten. Pause and repeat. Progress to "walking out" until the ball is under your ankles. On the ground, lie on your stomach, bend your knees (feet off the ground), and push up keeping the back flat.

Pushups on the Physioball. Walk out on the ball until the ball is under your knees.

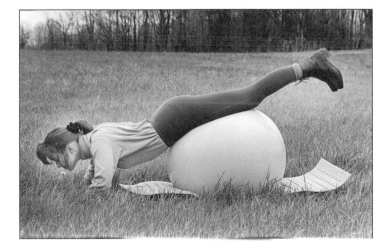

Perform a typical pushup, taking care to keep the back still. Progress to walking out until the ball meets your ankles. Repeat.

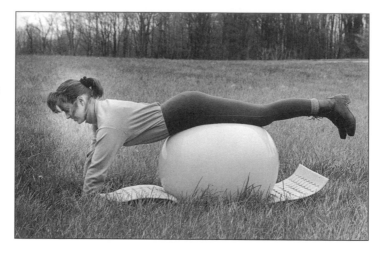

3. Upper Body

Seated Pulleys: Sit on the ball and secure an elastic Theraband around an object. Hold the Theraband like the reins. Squeezing your shoulder blades together, pull your elbows back just as you would exaggerate in reining back. Repeat the action and slowly release in sets of ten, adding increased resistance as the exercise becomes easier.

Mid-Back Strengthening. Sit on the Physioball and secure an elastic Theraband around an object. Hold the Theraband like the reins. Squeezing your shoulder blades together, pull your elbows back just as you would in reining back. Repeat the action and slowly release back to the starting position.

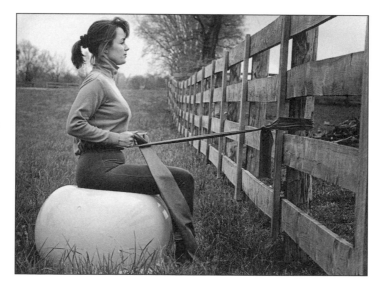

Rotator Cuff Strengthening: Seated, elbow at side, pull elastic band out as if opening a door. Slowly release. Repeat in sets of ten.

Rotator Cuff Strengthening. Seated, elbows at your side, pull the Theraband out as if opening a door.

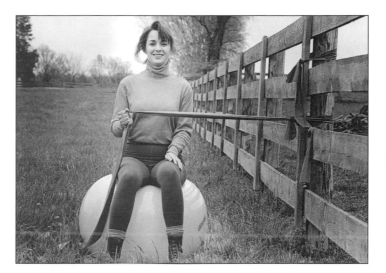

Slowly release the Theraband and repeat as for the Rotator Cuff.

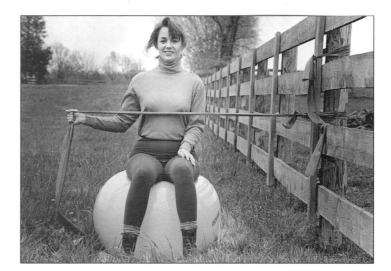

4. Lower Body

Partial Squats: Place your feet about hips' distance apart. Feet should face forward, much like they would be in the stirrups. Keeping the upper body in good alignment, lower your body down until your knees are at about a 90-degree angle. Hold the position for five seconds, then straighten the legs and raise the body. Repeat the movement in sets of ten, adding weights to the arms to lift as the exercise becomes easy. *Note: Don't perform a deep knee bend beyond 90 degrees as it can irritate the anterior knee.*

Partial Squats. Place your feet about hips' distance apart, feet facing forward as if you were in the saddle. Lower your body until your knees are at a 90-degree angle. Hold the position for five seconds, then slowly rise up. Repeat.

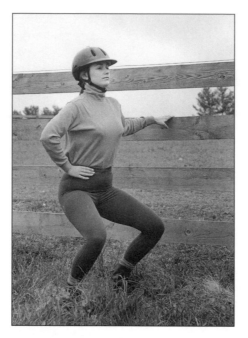

Riding-Specific Exercises

1. Hunt Seat/Endurance

All of the muscles of the lower body and trunk are used while a rider is in the two-point position. As previously mentioned, the lower body is a closed chain when our feet are in the stirrups. In hunt seat riding and endurance, the seat is raised out of the saddle, which causes our leg and back muscles to work harder to keep us in the saddle. To strengthen these muscles, I have incorporated the use of the Physioball to simulate the position of a rider and the three-dimensional movement of the horse.

Straddle the ball, gently squeezing the ball between your legs. Maintain the same aligned position you would assume in two-point. Simulate the jumping position by folding your upper body forward with your arms out in front of you. Be careful not to let your shoulders or upper back round, so only fold down as far as you can control. This becomes easier with practice and repetition. To add more challenge, have a friend attempt to push or pull you off balance, much like a horse might. Repeat this exercise in sets of ten. Add the resistance as needed.

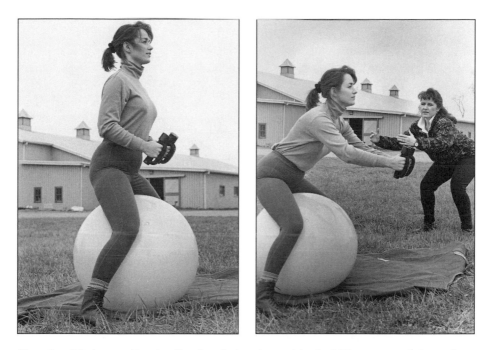

Hunt Seat/ Endurance Exercise. Simulate the jumping position by folding your trunk forward with your arms out in front of your body. Be careful not to let your shoulders or upper back round. To learn added control to maintain your position, have a friend jostle you and try to make you "dismount."

2. Dressage

Dressage requires good flexibility throughout the lower body, particularly the hip joint and lower back. Good lumbopelvic control is essential.

To practice the "pelvic motion," sit on the floor or on the exercise ball. Place one hand on the lower abdomen, the other hand in the small of the back. Tighten the abdominal muscles and feel that the lower back is flattening. Relax. Now contract the back muscle by pushing your tailbone down; note that the lower back arches. Repeat this motion until you can control a smooth and controlled rocking-type motion. Make sure you isolate the movement to the lower back to avoid compensating movements of the upper or lower body. Doing this exercise in front of a mirror is very helpful. Note: This is not a riding technique, but an exercise to make you more aware of your own movement and gain coordination and understanding of the motion.

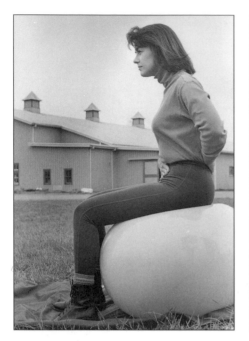

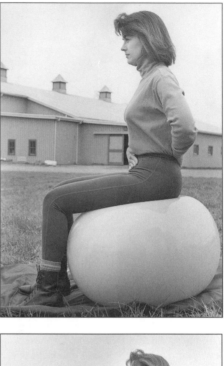

Dressage Exercise. Practice the "pelvic motion" seated on the Physioball. Place one hand on the lower abdomen, the other hand in the small of the back. Tighten the abdominals and feel the lower back flatten. Relax. Now contract the back muscle by sticking your tailbone down into the ball. Note that the lower back arches. Repeat these two motions until you can control a smooth rocking-type motion. Make sure you are isolating these exercises to the lower body and not including the upper body in your movements.

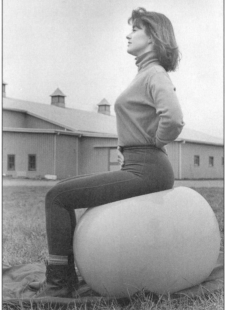

3. Western

Generally, western equitation requires flexibility similar to that of the dressage rider. Rodeo activities are quite different. For example, barrel racing and roping require trunk stability. Exercises such as the lean back featured here assist the rider in controlling the trunk similar to what is required for the more active disciplines.

Kneel on the floor or straddle the exercise ball. Tighten the abdominal and buttock muscles. Keeping the trunk absolutely still, lean back as far as you can maintain control. Hold the position for five seconds (isometrically contracting the muscles). Return to the upright position. Repeat in sets of ten.

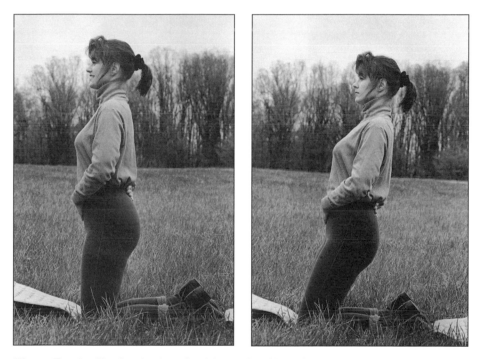

Western Exercise. Kneel and tighten the abdominal and buttock muscles. Keeping the trunk absolutely still, lean back as far as you can and still maintain control. Hold the position for a few seconds and return to the upright position.

4. Polo

Many women are now enjoying the traditionally male-dominated sport of polo. This sport requires a lot of balance and lower body strength as well as upper body flexibility and strength. To simulate aspects of the sport I have again incorporated the ball and the Theraband in the exercise.

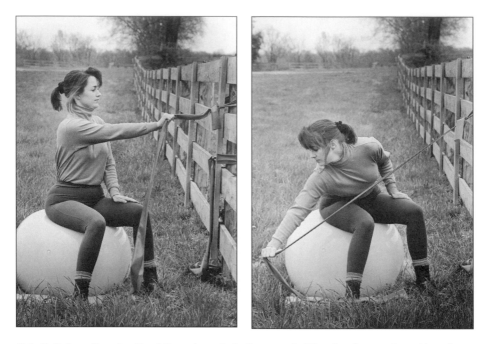

Polo Pull-down Exercise. Straddle or sit on the ball; secure the Theraband around an object. Grasp the Theraband and perform a series of bending motions toward one foot. Then pull the band up and across the body (similar to swinging the mallet with a backhand stroke).

Polo Pull-up Exercise. Grasp the Theraband and pull from your side, up and across your body (similar to swinging the mallet for a forehand shot).

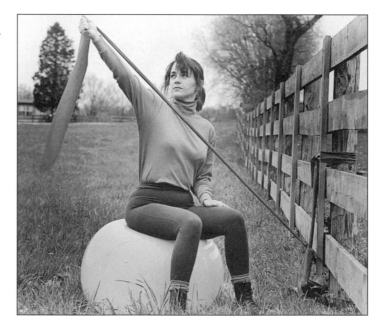

Straddle or sit on the exercise ball and secure the Theraband around a solid object. Grasp the Theraband and perform a series of bending motions toward one foot, then pull the band up and across the body as if hitting the mallet backhand. Conversely, grasp the Theraband and pull from your side up and across your body, as if hitting the mallet with a forward hand. Repeat the movements, going through a deeper range of motion as you gain control of the resistance.

5. Vaulting

Vaulting is essentially gymnastics on horseback. Therefore, performing gymnastic movements off and on the horse is at the heart of preparation and performance. It is not the intention of this book to review the various aspects of vaulting. However, cross-training with a vaulting lesson will help a rider develop her sense

AWAREness

The sooner you address a problem, the quicker you'll be in the saddle again enjoying a more comfortable ride.

A Quick Ten-Step Pre-ride Warm-Up Series

Take a few minutes and a deep breath before you get into the saddle. Throw a towel, saddle blanket or cooler on the ground and get started.

1. Calf stretch (page 86): Hold each leg for ten seconds and repeat.
2. Quad stretch (page 81): Hold each leg for ten seconds and repeat.
3. Side bend (page 89): ten repetitions on each side.
4. Standing hamstring stretch (page 82): Hold each leg for ten seconds and repeat.
5. Inner thigh stretch (page 84): Hold for ten seconds and repeat.
6. Piriformis stretch (page 85): Hold each leg for ten seconds.
7. Knees to chest, lower back stretch (page 86): Hold for ten seconds and repeat.
8. Prone press up (page 87): Hold for ten seconds and repeat.
9. Pectoral stretch (page 91): Hold for ten seconds and repeat.
10. Iliopsoas stretch: (page 82): Hold each leg for ten seconds and repeat.

of balance, body awareness and control. For further information, you might want to consult the references listed in the bibliography.

Exercise is useful for everyone. These exercises have assisted many of the riders Mary Beth has worked with in recovering from injuries, preventing injuries and en-hancing their performance. However, you might have a condition that would preclude performing some of these exercises. I encourage any rider with any concerns to have a full "pre-season" physical examination by her physician prior to engaging in physical activity.

Indications that medical attention is appropriate include any recurring muscle strain or spasm; ongoing pain in a joint, lower back or neck; or tingling sensations in any of the extremities. All of the above could be the result of a minor strain or a more serious condition, such as a herniated disc. Whatever the case, it is best to seek medical attention before the situation worsens.

Chapter 7

For Your Health and Safety

Although she may ride in good form, and, when her horse goes quietly, feel at home in the saddle, no woman can be considered proficient until she is prepared for any emergency, and knows how to meet it.—Elizabeth Karr, *The American Horsewoman,* 1884

Safety is the foundation of enjoyment. From another angle, lack of basic safety is a surefire way to ruin a riding experience, and possibly your life. Safety must be at the forefront of everyone's mind when working around, riding or driving horses. These are big animals capable of doing serious harm, unwittingly or on purpose. What we do with them—an athletic event, often at high speed—further increases the capacity for problems if we aren't reasonably careful.

That doesn't mean precaution has to impede the excitement of your sport or activity. It means that you can truly enjoy yourself if you properly lay the groundwork for a safe experience.

It is amazing to me how careless and unsafe horse people can be when compared to participants in other sports and recreational pursuits. Generally speaking, horses represent freedom to many people, and those same people may have a tendency to disregard safety in the pursuit of that freedom. On a positive note, technology has finally found some openings into the horse world, and new products and improvements appear every day.

Tradition and technology aside, it all starts with you and some common sense. As coordinator and a board member of Markel Corporation's Markel Equestrian Safety

Board (MESB), I am very aware of safety issues for the equestrian and the horse. Recently, the MESB established the following minimum national safety guidelines for participants in horse sports.

Minimum Safety Guidelines for Participants

- Develop a basic understanding of horse behavior and inherent risks.

- Follow established safety guidelines at your riding facility and at horse-related events.

- Wear protective headgear and proper footwear and clothing.

- Inspect and maintain tack and equipment regularly.

- Maintain physical fitness and health comparable to the demands of your horse activity.

Understanding Horse Behavior

People who are getting started with horses should learn as much as possible about them and their behavior. Usually, that means getting as much experience as possible with the animal itself. Some of us live on farms, and others may be city-based, but the requirement is the same: Get to know the animal. Horses are a never-ending learning process. There will always be surprises, but being aware of what can happen is half the battle when it comes to safety and injury prevention.

Consider these observations based on my own experience:

Horses are prey and herd animals designed to live in a veritable caste system. Some are dominant and some submissive, and pecking orders are established early in their lives. Their basic behavioral characteristics are related to survival. In a barn or farm situation, your horse will fit into a niche, which can help explain some of his behavior toward you. Pay attention to your horse's field and barn behavior.

Know and understand the behavior of the sexes. Mares, geldings and stallions all have their own distinctive patterns. Pick up an animal behavior book, take a class or have an informal discussion about it with a professional. It is very important that you try to understand the natural instincts that are driving your horse. Remember they are in tune with nature; we brought them into our world.

Generally speaking, fillies and mares are much more sensitive than males about their hindquarters, and are quicker to tuck and kick out for protection. If you think about it, that makes sense: In the wild, they are protecting themselves from being mounted and signaling to the male they are not ready to breed. On the other hand, males and even geldings can become excited by the simple presence of a mare, especially if they are separated most of the time, and their behaviors are often very obviously dictated by interest in a female.

AWAREness

Most "bad" behavior comes from a clash between the innate instincts of the horse and the rules we humans are imposing on it.

I learned my lesson the hard way once when I rode my mare into a field of geldings. All of the cross-country jumps happened to be in their field and I thought we could jump in one area while the geldings quietly grazed at the other end. Even though the field was quite large, I was taking my life into my hands, as I soon found out. I have seen the reverse to be true as well, when mares have challenged an unfamiliar male intruder.

In addition to mating, food is a basic survival instinct. If, for instance, you go out into a field of horses with a bucket of feed, you will quickly see their system of survival in action. If you pay attention, you can see a sense of order to it. They may rush toward you at first, but by talking to them as you approach (or they approach you), the process organizes itself around you. The horses that are most dominant will position themselves by nipping, biting, kicking or wheeling to get to the feed first. If your horse is not one of these dominant types, you may have a difficult time navigating toward him while others circle around you. You have to feel your way through the situation as well—you could be getting into the middle of a social riot or a stampede, in which case you have to remove yourself from the scene calmly but purposefully. I've been in the middle of a few of these.

Whenever possible and practical, take someone out to the field with you, work together as a team and communicate. Be as calming as possible. If your horse is difficult to catch without an incentive, one of you should be prepared to offer small handfuls of feed or some carrots while the other puts a halter and lead rope on your horse. If you have to go alone, take your time and don't make any startling moves. Just be aware that anything can stir horses to move as one very powerful group. It is this situation, the group startle, that can cause serious commotion and create a safety issue for you.

Gates can produce particular behaviors, notably pushing and shoving, because horses associate them with activities that happen on the other side (feeding, grooming and so forth). I like to carry a white wand (T.T.E.A.M.) along with me so that when I open the gate, I can tap—never whip or use quick movements— horses out of the way and stroke them to calm them down. This allows me to establish some distance at first but also acts as an extension of me that is firm but not threatening enough to spook them. Yelling and screaming will only get them more revved up: "An angry word will raise a horse's pulse to an extraordinary degree. He has a very keen ear for what is conveyed by the tone of the voice and manner of speaking" (*Modern Side-Saddle Riding,* 1907).

When turning out a horse, exercise caution. The horse's natural tendency is to run into a field (whether or not you are completely ready to release him), and by anticipating this behavior you can avoid a problem. You go through the gate first, and while you are holding the gate in one hand, watch the horse go through and make sure he doesn't catch a shoulder or hip. Once in the field, turn the horse back toward you and the gate and stand quietly, thereby counteracting his natural impulse to run out. If your horse has a tendency to bolt when you let him loose, stand with him for an extra long period of time and stroke him. You may even want to latch the gate and walk a distance into the field, but always turn the horse toward you and the gate before you set him free. Slowly unlatch the halter and slip it off. If the horse stands with you for a moment when free, reward him. Do not yell or wave at him to go away. Let your horse leave you first, then return and secure the gate.

(I strongly recommend that horses be turned out without halters. If you have a horse that is very difficult to catch and you feel the need to keep the halter on, make sure the halter fits properly so that he won't get hung up in trees or on fences or get a leg through a noseband that is too loose. I've seen and heard of some very unfortunate events related to halters.)

Body Position and Spatial Considerations

Body position is a means of communication between horses. Not surprisingly, the horse interprets and takes cues from your body position as well. To be safe around horses, you have to be aware of this and move within some well-defined parameters. If you don't, you could take a relatively serene situation and turn it into a safety problem.

AWAREness

If you take time to recognize and understand the horse's natural tendencies, you can anticipate events and situations that test safety.

Your horse should have been trained to lead properly as a youngster. If not, consult a professional to teach him to lead. You will want to be there so you can be a part of the experience. You and your horse need to learn this together.

The most usual nonriding activity you and your horse are involved in is moving from place to place, when you are leading him around. Here are safety tips to keep in mind about this deceptively simple activity:

- When leading a horse, don't wrap the lead rope around your hand, arm or any part of your body. Make large loops in the excess and carry them with an open hand. Hold onto the fabric or leather part of the lead, not the clasp.

- Position yourself between the middle of the horse's neck and shoulder area and learn to turn him. The most advantageous way to turn a horse is away from you so that you don't get stepped on or have body weight pressed against you. You should remain at the mid-neck to shoulder area at all times. If you are in a tight spot and can't turn the horse away, bring him toward you by holding the lead in your left hand, and with your right hand, gently push on his ribs to move him away in the rear and toward you in the front.

    When you want to stop and secure the horse, how you do it is important. Quick-release tying is a basic safety precaution. Have a professional show you how to tie a quick-release knot. You will use it daily and at shows and can feel secure in knowing both you and your horse are out of harm's way if danger occurs. Always tie your horse to a very solid and smooth surface. Look around the area and imagine what he can get into if you have to leave momentarily.

Most stables use cross-ties to secure horses for grooming or tacking up. Cross-ties are convenient and give you room to maneuver in a clear aisle on a hard clean surface. If I had my choice, however, I would prefer to see a quick release tie to a wall in the aisle or wash stall or inside the horse's stall for safety purposes. Cross-ties offer no safe escape if and when a horse panics, and they all do. When a horse breaks through cross-ties they can damage themselves by wrenching or straining neck and back muscles, misalign a vertebrae or throw their entire body out of alignment. They can also cause chaos in the aisle and possibly injure people and other horses, not to mention run away.

The quick release option gives you a fast, safe way to save you and your horse. It's another smart form of risk management.

The way you handle your horse and the body language you employ will determine whether or not your horse is tense. If he is, the odds of something dangerous happening increase. The manner in which you respond to a horse's anxiety can also help to defuse a potentially difficult situation.

An anxious or high-strung horse may be calmed using a technique I have found successful. One of the ways horses manifest their tension is in their necks, where tightness can signal upset. A rocking motion can help release energy from the base of the neck, essentially breaking up tension. The exercise described below is great for quieting a horse at a show, and also for warming up before mounting. Peggy Cummings taught this technique to me, and some of her clients use it regularly in the vet box at three-day events. I wish I had known about it years ago when I was preparing yearlings for the sales. I would love to see racehorse handlers adopt this method; it would eliminate a lot of horse and human stress and injuries.

Calming the Anxious Horse

This can be accomplished on either side of the horse when leading. First, make sure the halter or bridle is properly fitted and not loose or dangling. It is important to have a close fit around the nose so that the horse's head can be moved in a supporting way. Stand on the horse's left side and put the lead line through the noseband ring closest to you. Weave the lead line in through the ring down, then up across the nose continuing in the ring on the other side to come out and hook on the top ring with the snap button away from horse. Hold the lead in your left hand and slide your right hand, four fingers together with a flat hand, under the noseband (take all of the slack out of the lead). The back of your hand should be flat against the horse's muzzle. Now close your hand so you have the noseband firmly in hand. You can do this with just a halter, but the halter must be fairly snug or you won't have a handle to work with. You now have control of the horse's head and can move it away from you and toward you.

If you are working with the bridle, slip the reins over the head and hold them in your left hand. Slide your right hand, four fingers together, with a flat hand under the noseband at the T junction of the cheek piece. The back of your hand should be flat against the horse's muzzle. Close your hand so that you have the noseband firmly in hand.

The object is to work with a soft arm to move the horse's head while he's walking and teach the horse that the poll can release while walking (like patting your head and rubbing your stomach). Sometimes it takes six or eight strides and you feel the horse let go and soften. Other times it takes a small circle (10 to 12 meters) and walking the horse in S patterns throughout the circle to encourage a release. The important thing is to be encouraging without pushing and pulling and to remain soft in your arms and hands.

Teaching the horse to release at the poll while walking in a non-habitual way helps the horse release the body and focus on a rhythm engaging thought rather than reaction.

In the beginning the back-and-forth motion is larger but once the horse has released the oscillation is imperceptible. This is a soothing exercise for you and your horse.

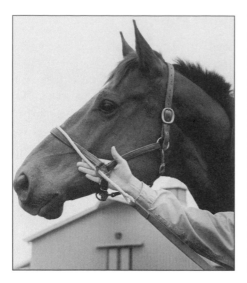

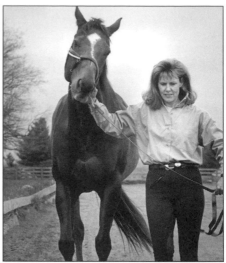

To help calm an anxious or head-high horse, begin by placing your hand under the noseband and clasping the noseband and lead line. The noseband should be snug and properly placed on the face.

You are now ready to begin the walking-and-rocking motion. Ask the horse to move on by pushing his head slightly away from you and back toward you again. Repeat this motion and allow him to take the first step. In other words, don't drag him into the walk.

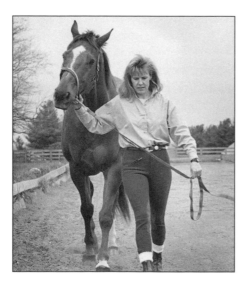

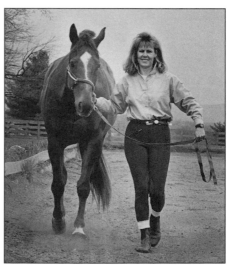

As you walk, bring his head toward you, back to center and away from you. Once you begin walking and rocking, it should become a rhythmical, smooth motion.

If the horse resists or continues to go head-high, keep the motion going—jiggle or vibrate your hand and try to break up the tension in an S pattern or by circling 10 to 12 meters.

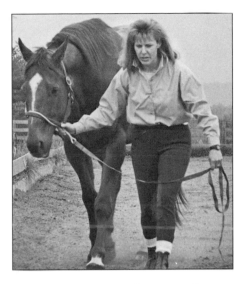

As the horse's head comes down, move down with him by keeping your knees bent. This encourages him to relax even more.

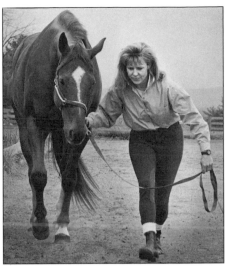

Once a horse has experienced this technique, he usually remembers it and relaxes with only a few walking steps.

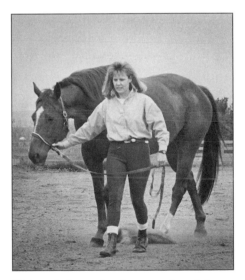

Ultimately, horses that have experienced the rocking-and-walking motion calm down more readily and you have less warmup time and a lot less stress.

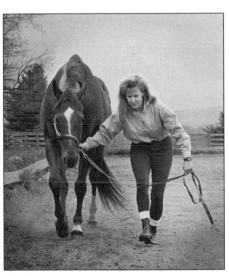

Now, Kippy's Surprise is relaxed and listening to me. We both can have an enjoyable opportunity.

Keeping Yourself Sound

Intelligent horse care is made up of a series of activities and choices, many of which we take for granted or don't completely think through before we act. Consider these cautionary observations about life with horses.

Around the Barn

1. Use a hose to water each stall; when buckets are low or empty, carry them to the water source for cleaning. If you have to cart water, use a wheelbarrow or buy a small wagon for hauling around the barn.

2. Carry and haul as little as possible. Get a friend to help you. Serve feed and hay from a wheelbarrow. To cart equipment back and forth, use a tack trunk with wheels, a hand truck (dolly) or a wheelbarrow.

3. Small women, this one's for you: You need to minimize reaching up when grooming, blanketing, and tacking up. This may sound impossible, but you should know that by reaching up all the time to work around and on the horse, you are using poor body mechanics that likely will result in damage over time. You'll be paid back in pain. And don't be talked into buying a 17-hand horse. It only puts stress and strain on your body.

    If you have to work with tall horses, purchase a lightweight stool (look for width and stability) at any hardware or home goods store. Use it around your horse as much as possible, being careful to plant it securely on level ground. This is good for blanketing, braiding, pulling manes, grooming heads and backs, bridling, and placing saddles and pads correctly. And if you do a lot of massage work like I do, it's great for getting adequate pressure on the back, croup and tail-head areas. Without elevation, your grooming is ineffective and you will experience inflamed shoulders and a tight neck. Once you are elevated, not only will your currying and brushing techniques improve, your muscles and joints will be lined up correctly for the task at hand. Your chores will be toning instead of damaging your body.

4. Incorporate proper body mechanics into your daily chores no matter what your size.

> **AWAREness**
>
> *Put yourself in the right position to achieve the right outcome.*

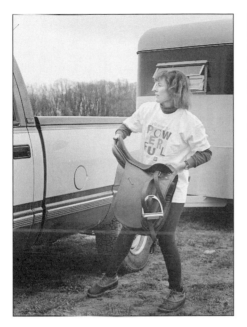

Leslie Wood hoists her saddle into the truck.

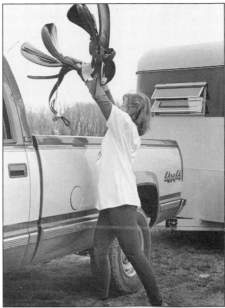

Poor biomechanics at work. Every muscle in Leslie's upper body is being abused.

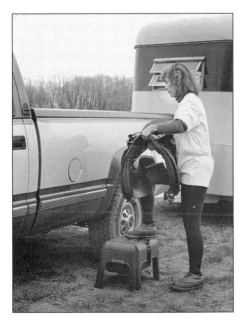

Now Leslie carries a stool in her truck so that she can use her strong legs and lower back to lift heavy objects.

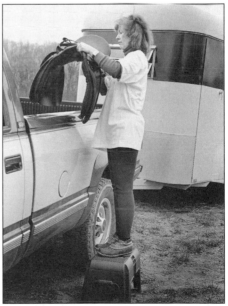

Relate the biomechanics of this picture to everything you do around your horse and the barn. Using the correct biomechanics and a stool can make a great deal of difference in how comfortable you will be later on.

In Training

1. Try to be as ambidextrous as possible. It will help tremendously in your riding and in-hand/ground work. Train your horse from both sides equally to give both of you effective conditioning. Forget about doing everything from the left. That custom was established centuries ago for reasons of convenience and aesthetics. Nowadays, we're talking about two athletes working together to achieve balance. Try to conduct your leading, ground and mounted training work on both sides. (This is especially important in retraining a racehorse that always competed with the rail on his left. The right side of his body is likely to be underdeveloped and unaware of how to bend and flex.)

2. Teach young horses to lead without pulling or pressure. They need to be taught to "think" at an early age. The TT.E.A.M. approach is the most effective method I have found for accomplishing this. You will appreciate this training later on when the horse is 1,100 pounds instead of a more manageable 600 pounds and under 15 hands.

AWAREness

For any discipline or use, horses built "downhill" or "pullers" such as ex-racehorses, can be hard on women's shoulders and backs. They often require longer warm-ups and training sessions, causing greater wear and tear on you and themselves.

3. Learn riding methods that promote self-carriage and relaxation in the horse. (See chapter 4.) Your horse and your body will appreciate the consideration and riding will remain a positive experience throughout your life.

4. Select a horse that matches your ability, temperament, personality and size. Take time to write out a job description when you are horse shopping and act as though you are conducting an interview. You're the boss looking for a new partner in success. What are the qualifications? What won't you accept? Which one would you hire to complement you? If you are buying with the guidance of a professional trainer, work out the description together.

5. Select a horse that is built for your sport. The form-to-function lesson is operative here.

6. Girls and women should select a horse that offers a more "uphill" or balanced conformation. This type of body build will tend to minimize heavy-on-the-forehand or "pulling" problems that greatly add to women's shoulder and back pain and injury. The older I get, the more experienced I am as a rider, the more I look for "uphill" horses.

Dressing to Ride

Protective Headgear

Rule Number One: Never mount a horse without protective headgear. It's that simple.

Thirty people a day are admitted to emergency rooms in the United States with head injuries related to equestrian accidents.[1] That makes 10,000 riders a year! And we don't know how many never even make it to the emergency room. Why take the chance? It's your life that's at stake.

As long as you are smart, take responsibility for your own quality of life and protect yourself. Horses are fun and the best recreational and sporting activity around. Without protection, riding can be one of the highest-risk activities known. So many professionals believe they are immune to the danger because they are experienced. Experience has nothing to do with the laws of physics and probability: Accidents are going to happen. Whether you are sitting on a horse or jumping at top speed, a similar amount of risk exists. That may be hard to believe and understand, but the injury data prove it.

I try to take the time to educate the unhelmeted, even if it does produce the occasional uncomfortable moment.

[1] This estimate is derived from the 1990–92 National Electronic Injury Surveillance System (NEISS) recreational injury survey. The National Consumer Product Safety Commission oversees the survey and records injuries reported by hospital emergency rooms and from these figures gives national projections of injuries.

Riders no longer have an excuse for not wearing a safety helmet. In particular, the longstanding complaints of women are now being addressed by designs that answer our needs. For example, Troxel Equestrian is designing helmets with elements women appreciate. Troxel's protective headgear is lightweight (eleven ounces—you can't even tell there's anything in the box when you buy it); well ventilated for maximum air flow, which will help prevent against heat stress, disorientation and masked judgments; and adjustable, using a customized padding system to fit the shape and size of your head. The headgear also features a Pony Tail Port so you don't lose integrity in the fit; has a safety retention system so the helmet stays on your head (important when you are falling); and is made with a thin micro-shell that meets the highest safety standards and fits more snugly against your head (no more pumpkin-head). These helmets even help avoid "hat hair!"

AWAREness

Those who fail to protect themselves increase their own risk and the liability the rest of us pay for in the form of insurance premiums. Other people not wearing helmets is our business.

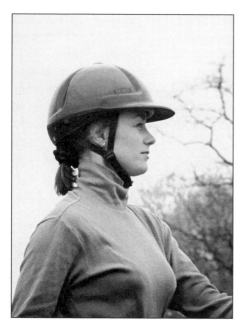

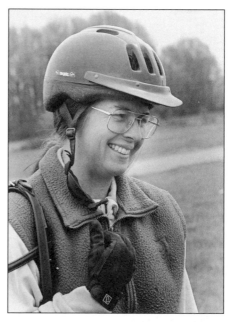

Gwyn Donohue is wearing Troxel's "Legacy" helmet, which meets ASTM/SEI safety requirements and features a "Pony Tail Port."

Alice Magaha, Western and English trainer and instructor, prepares to snap on the chin strap of her Troxel "Sport" helmet, which meets ASTM/SEI safety requirements.

Always wear a helmet that meets the ASTM/SEI (American Society for Testing Materials/Safety Equipment Institute) safety standards. Every day, manufacturers are designing helmets that meet these safety standards, meet the needs of our sport, meet the needs of women in particular, and are simply a lot more attractive.

The western disciplines have yet to embrace or recommend protective headgear. If you are involved in western, you should at least wear a schooling helmet when you are at home and warming up at the show. Slip on your Stetson before you go into the show ring. There are lightweight, well ventilated helmets on the market that meet the highest safety standards. It will take a great deal of self-confidence to wear one when your peers aren't, but rest assured that *everyone* will be sooner or later. Be the smart one and protect yourself starting today. You'll live to tell your children about it.

Reasonable head protection that looks good is the wave of the future. If nothing else, we are being forced toward safety because of the legal ramifications of being unsafe. Wearing protective headgear will become mandatory in our lifetime. The sooner it happens, the better it will be for safety-conscious riders who will no longer have to carry the burden of costs for the injuries and irresponsibility of others. Many states have passed laws that require cyclists to wear helmets, and laws that affect riders similarly will not be too far behind unless we take it upon ourselves to do the right thing.

Build your personal safety program with a helmet. Today.

How to Fit a Helmet

The helmet fits when it is level front to back and the front edge extends down to about an inch from the top of the eyebrows. The helmet should fit snugly and should not slide freely about the head. When properly adjusted, the helmet should not "roll" forward or backward. It should not be removable without unbuckling the strap.

For your helmet size, carefully run a measuring tape around the circumference of your head, about one inch above the eyebrows, front to back.

A 1993 study [2] indicates that women's heads are shaped differently from men's, and on the average, shorter from front to back. While the female head is wider (in proportion to its length) than that of the male, the actual area is smaller.

Many helmets have not been designed in consideration of women's sizing. Look for the ones with accommodation for hair (ponytails) and a custom fit for the variety in head size and shape.

Footwear

It is important for you to be protected in the saddle with proper footwear. Always wear a closed shoe or boot with a solid, flat heel. I prefer no laces on footwear; however, field and paddock boots with short laces are an acceptable exception. Sneakers and sandals, which I see a lot of in warm-up areas at horse shows, are totally unacceptable. Soft and toeless shoes can go through a stirrup very easily or bend when jammed forward (such as in a sudden stop) inside a closed stirrup (such as on a western saddle). This is not an issue of style or convenience—you need support and the heel for protection. Even when you are unmounted, solid foot-wear is important. You never know when you may get stepped on.

Clothing for the Rider

Dress for riding with these four things in mind:

1. Weather

2. Fit

3. Comfort

4. Activity

Layering

The principal challenge in dressing for riding lies in the temperature extremes that we face. Beside the obvious difference between winter and summer, we are often faced with dramatic changes in a day or even in a morning, when

[2]Anthropometry of the Head and Face in Medicine (Dreyfuss Associates).

a barn that has been refrigerated overnight turns into an oven within hours. And in our work and riding, some moments are active and some are not.

Layering is an answer. Wearing several layers, all designed for outdoor and sport activities, allows you to adjust as your body temperature moves from its coldest state while standing around to the hottest while working your horse or grooming. At stake is your health: Excessive physical activity when you are cold and underdressed leads directly to strained muscles; exertion when you are hot and overdressed leads directly to fatigue, exhaustion, mental mistakes and accidents.

Keep in mind that you are working just as hard as your horse. It is up to you to hold up your end of the partnership with a cool, protected head and a body that is dressed for the task at hand. Your appearance, even at the barn, says a lot about you, most notably whether you are a safe and intelligent rider.

Search the catalogs and sporting goods and tack stores for new materials designed for sport activities. The technology is out there and new materials for sporting activities come on the market every day. There are tremendous crossover opportunities for multisport clothing use. Use your imagination.

The following sequence of considerations, from the inside out, offers you a way to think through the issue of clothes and riding.

Undergarments are the most important layer You should be wearing a sports bra that fits and supports you properly and moves with your activity. It is most helpful to wear a sports bra that can also be worn as an outer garment. Many of them come in neutral, bright colors and patterns. At shows, or when you have to change clothes, you can do so without seeking out a private area.

It is impossible to list all the bras currently on the market, but we have included some models to look for, depending on your breast size and what you feel is most comfortable. Essentially, athletic bras come in two styles— those that compress the breast close to the body to avoid jarring (best for women with smaller breasts) and those that lift and separate and hold the breasts in place.

A multicolored sports bra for larger-breasted women by Support Team for underwear or outerwear use.

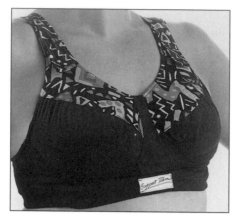

Every woman has her own opinion about what looks and feels good, but when you are shopping for a bra you should be able to jump around the dressing room without jumping out of your bra or causing excessive movement of the breasts. Whatever you choose, the bra should be comfortable, nonrestrictive and give you the best possible figure.

Common sense suggests that you don't reach for your sexy underpants to ride. Frilly, delicate underwear may look great, but it is not functional for sports and certainly not comfortable for riding. Go for comfort, padding and no seams. Several brands of underwear are especially made for long hours in the saddle. Look for material that wicks away perspiration and encourages air flow. It's important to protect your genital area from saddle sores and chafing. Keep the glamour on the outside and stay protected underneath.

The next layer of clothing should be made of a lightweight, wicking material Check out sporting goods stores or catalogs for the latest materials designed to keep you dry and comfortable.

Moving Comfort (a Springfield, Virginia, company owned by two women, one of whom rides regularly) produces active wear for women that makes sense for our activities and our bodies. You can wear their clothes for running one day, riding the next—a great choice for those of us into cross-training. These products will keep you dry and comfortable underneath heavier clothing in the

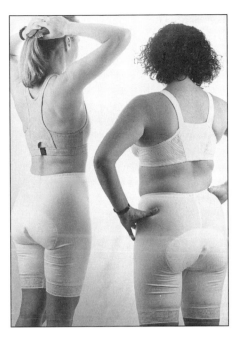

No matter what your size, you should be prepared to ride with the proper undergarments year-round. Pictured, "Cover Your Assets" underwear by Equi-Logic.

winter and well-ventilated during the summer. The models in the exercise photographs are wearing this company's clothing.

Breeches, tights, pants, or jeans should be seamless through the crotch area and preferably have a side closure Seamless garments will decrease any friction or binding that might occur. The inside of your knees should be protected from chafing and the ankle area should be secured to prevent these garments from wrinkling or riding up when you are mounted.

Outer clothes should be fairly close-fitting without being tight Scarves and jewelry are absolutely out. Once you've seen someone hook a scarf, necklace, ring, bracelet or earring on or around a horse or equipment, you'll never think of wearing them again. I typically wear a sports watch made of plastic or rubber, my wedding band and tiny, smooth post earrings.

Wear socks that keep your feet dry in any season Dry feet are a key source of good feeling and a good gauge of how well we've prepared. When our feet are dry we are usually comfortable.

When showing, keep collars, stock ties and ratcatchers (or chokers) fairly loose around your neck and wrists   Your stress level and nerves are up, and you're probably perspiring regardless of the weather. You need to stay cool and keep the air flow moving. Dickeys are excellent for adding the show look without adding more bulk and weight under your jacket.

Equipment Safety

Your horse is a dynamic, changing animal. Check your equipment for proper fit often. The equipment we use must be selected with the animal's environment and natural movement in mind.

Your horse's body changes just as yours does—up and down with the seasons, work load, age, type of feed, stress levels and so on. When your horse is out of work or on grass, he will look very different than when fit and on grain. Muscle tone and development are a direct corollary of work and diet. The horse's frame also changes when you are competing, riding more regularly or changing sports—say from fast work on trails to arena work. Constantly check for these changes and how your equipment fits with the development.

Balance, control and comfort are as important to the horse's performance as they are to your riding.

For maximum safety, check your tack for repair and cleanliness. If you are buying tack, used or new, check out the stitching, the seams and the face of the leather or nylon for age and cracking. Before you buy, ask the tack store about its policy on guaranteeing a sound saddle tree.

Salt, saliva, sweat and dirt are corrosive to leather. This is the major reason why many endurance riders have chosen alternatives to leather for their tack to combat these corrosive elements and achieve low maintenance. Keep a clean, soft sponge available for tack only. At the very least, wipe your equipment down after every use. If you keep your tack properly maintained and check the integrity of the equipment regularly, you're on your way to riding safely.

The Bridle

You probably pay more attention to your saddle and girth than other equipment. Take your bridle home and clean it thoroughly often. You can sit on the floor in front of the television at night with some newspaper and a small bucket of warm, soapy water and completely disassemble it. If you have kids, get them involved, but don't let the dog think it's a new rawhide.

While your bit is soaking, give all of the cheek pieces, browband, noseband, reins, etc., a thorough cleaning with a high-quality saddle soap and warm water. If you have time or you're preparing to show, you go a step further and polish the brass and silver fittings. Once you've put the bridle back together, remembering the proper holes for the fit (you can use masking tape as markers for new equipment), figure-eight the reins through the throatlatch and hang it up by the headstall. Leave it by the front door and you're ready to go the next day.

Stirrups

Stirrups are a real safety concern and a key part of your equipment. The type of riding you do doesn't matter. Whether English or Western, choose a product for safety. There are many on the market today. With an eye on new developments, don't ignore the basics: Make sure stirrups have properly fitted pads or gripping material to avoid slippage, especially when wet. New, very strong, lightweight materials are being introduced with safety design qualities for stirrups.

Pads, Wraps and Rugs

Make sure your saddle pads and wraps are clean and debris-free. If you use equipment made from rope, cotton, lambswool, nylon, string or other materials, check for loose threads and connections to metal or leather. Most of the ones made today can be washed in a machine and hung up to dry. The integrity of the material is what you need to keep your eye on. Sweat and dirt will wear these products down too.

Many horse people (and in my experience, usually women) have become turnout-rug crazy. Generally, the motives for "over-rugging" a horse are not particularly commendable: Riders don't want to deal with a long coat, cleanup, long cool-outs and so on, and the idea of lower maintenance in our busy schedules is attractive. This tradeoff is not likely to change, but there is a particular consequence to be avoided. In my travels, I see more and more jammed and sore shoulders and withers caused by ill-fitting blankets. Remember that they are human contraptions and a part of domesticating the horse. If you think of the hours horses spend with blankets on—blanket wearing takes up a major portion of their winter life and in some show stables they wear them year-round—you'll recognize that you mustn't shortchange this piece of equipment. Make sure your horse has plenty of freedom while wearing the blanket and choose one that comes up around the base of the neck instead of behind the withers where it can pull and rub on the chest, inhibiting movement and stretching. To prevent accidents, check for straps that hang too low or are twisted. Above all, if you are going to be using a blanket extensively, don't just look for the cheapest or prettiest model.

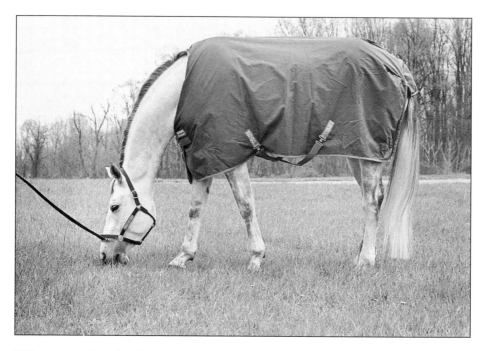

Make sure your horse has plenty of freedom while wearing a blanket. Choose one that comes up around the base of the neck instead of behind the withers, where it can pull and rub on the chest, cramp the shoulders and inhibit movement. Your horse lives in the grazing position even in the stall.

Now that your equipment is in good shape, educate yourself by learning from a professional how to properly fit a saddle, a stable sheet and a turnout blanket, and how to bandage or wrap your horse's legs. It is crucial that your equipment be properly fitted every time you use it.

A Guide to Saddle Fitting

Saddles are perhaps the prime example of equipment traditionally built for men, and as a consequence cause problems for female riders. There are also issues which apply to all riders, female and male, in the effort to incorporate safety into their approach to saddles. We can't cover every aspect of saddle fitting here, but we can provide you with information that will benefit you and your horse. (Photographs by Peggy Cummings unless otherwise indicated.)

Keep in mind that we are primarily discussing saddle *fitting* rather than saddle *buying*. Our objective is to create the best fit possible with what you already have. Manufacturers generally design saddles to fit a horse standing still. How often do horses stand still when we are riding? Hardly ever. Even when they do stand, they shift their weight around. Our goal is to fit equipment to work with a moving, changing, dynamic animal.

Background

Saddles are supported by the horse's bone structure, incorporating the ribs and thoracic vertebrae, and by the structure of the hind and fore limbs. An incorrectly positioned saddle can impede movement, especially shoulder and hind end movement. Saddles are also supported by large muscles that connect the other body areas. An ill-fitting saddle will reduce the function of these muscles:

- Head and neck muscle into back (trapezius)

- Foreleg muscle into back (latissimus dorsi)

- Balance coordination in gait (longissimus dorsi)

- Spinal muscle, ligaments and connective tissue

When bones or muscles are affected, overall performance of the horse is affected.

Saddles obviously also come into contact with the skin surface of the horse's back. A poorly fitted saddle will cause shutdown and damage to the skin tissue. When a saddle damages the skin, the overall health of the horse may be affected:

- Circulation (nutrient, blood supply, warming)
- Ventilation (cooling, heat loss)
- Perspiration (sweat cooling)
- Nerve network (sensitivity)
- Pressure points (healing, conditioning)
- Protective covering (hair and dermal layers)

Approach

For you and your horse, the fit of your saddle is crucial to your performance, and compensating for differences in your particular situation (horse, saddle and rider) is the key. In my mind, the best approach is to work from the horse itself. The saddle won't work unless it fits the horse, which is why I've prepared the following information to help you evaluate saddle fit from the standpoint of both you and your horse. Peggy Cummings and Steve Ray Gonzalez (an outstanding Bellingham, Washington–based saddle designer) provided me with important information.

Saddle Fitting Points

Mental Checklist

Keep the following points in mind:

1. Horses are changing and dynamic
2. Check the fit often as the seasons change and if the horse's work or nutritional regimen changes

Saddle Components

The saddle a rider sees and contacts is only the covering of the saddle's basic foundation. It is this foundation, or *saddle tree,* that dictates the physical connection between the rider and the horse. All saddles have a tree and contain the same basic elements:

Bars   Structures that are the foundation for the rider's seat and stirrup attachment.

Fork, Pommel or Head   The structure that offers the integrity of the saddle tree and sits near the withers.

Cantle   The structure that keeps the rider from sliding off the back of the saddle.

Seat   Supports the rider in a sitting position (a balance platform).

- Formed on the bars of the tree with the pommel at the front and the cantle at the rear.

- Proper seat shape provides for anatomically correct posture for the rider.

- Correct seat position on the tree will provide a proper balance platform for the rider and provide for proper weight placement and distribution to the horse.

Stirrups   Support the rider's weight in a standing position (a balance platform).

- Attached to bars of the saddle tree.

- Stirrup leathers and the position of the irons will dictate balance or imbalance of rider (first important element toward a balanced seat).

Rigging   Equipment for securing the saddle to the horse (billets, etc.).

- Position on the tree must match the natural girth position on the horse.

According to Steve Ray Gonzalez, "The proper function of a saddle can be accomplished when all the dimensions of the tree match the surface dimensions of the horse." In other words, a perfect match (or mold) of the saddle tree to the horse's back is the ideal. But, he adds, "Perfection is not necessary to achieve a functional fit." The objective is simply to get as close as possible to the ideal.

Saddle Function

Saddles must allow the natural movement of *both* horse and rider. When saddle tree dimensions do not match horse dimensions, the result is imbalance of horse and rider, reduced security for the rider, and injury to the horse from excessive pressure or friction on the back.

Considerations

1. Security: The saddle's physical structure provides a stronghold for the rider to the horse.

2. Balance/Centering Platform: The physical elements of the saddle provide a platform for the rider to center in posture and balance in performance.

   - Seat must be the right size and shape for you in order for it to act as a balancing platform.

   - Rise and angle of the waist (twist) of the saddle leading up to the pommel is greater for the female rider to support her pubic arch. (Look at the seat of your saddle and notice where the stitching narrows, as in a body's waist. Follow from there up to the pommel. This is the area that is markedly changed to fit the female pubic arch.)

3. Weight Distribution: The saddle provides the proper placement, distribution and transmission of the rider's weight and movements into the horse's body.

4. Positioning: Rider's weight should be evenly distributed between the horse's eighth and eighteenth ribs.

   - A horse's back can accept a maximum of 1.5 pounds per square inch without discomfort. Judge the area involved accordingly.

   - Contact of the saddle surface with the horse's back surface should be even. To check for even distribution, note sweat and dirt marks on your white saddle pad. The areas under the saddle that stay clean are not contacting the horse. Or sift a light coating of powder or flour on a dark horse's back and place your saddle carefully on it. Now lift straight up (you are standing on a stool to do this correctly, right?)

and notice where the saddle has and has not contacted the back.

5. Equine Center/Balance: A correctly functioning saddle will allow proper balance of the horse through all gaits and movements.

There is no contact between this saddle and the horse's back, as indicated by Peggy Cummings' hand.

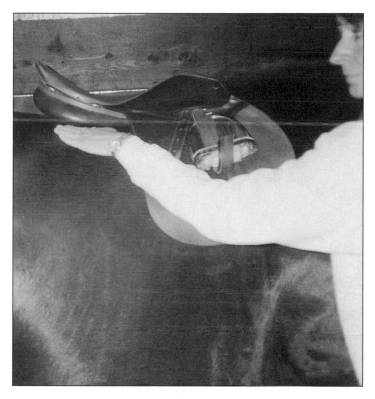

Proper Fit of Your Saddle

A proper saddle fit will give maximum function of the tree to the horse and rider. No saddle will fit every horse, and more importantly, some saddles may become unworkable because of changes in the horse (or rider). There may be situations where you might have to replace your saddle because you determine that the tree is too narrow, too long or too wide. A horse's back has limits as to what it will accept.

If you keep at it, you'll develop an "eye" for saddle fit. Focus first on the lowest point of the seat of the saddle to determine if it is level, and work from there.

At first glance, this may look like a good fit. But a closer look shows that the seat is too far back, causing an uphill battle for the rider. The horse's shoulders are being pinched, and there is a great deal of rigging to keep the saddle in place.

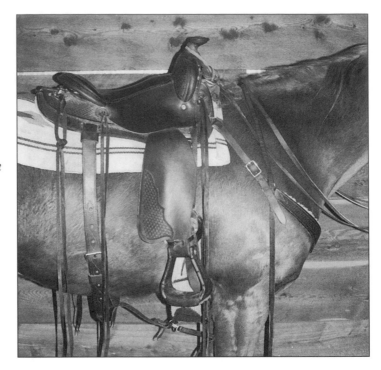

Identifying Poor Fit

1. Saddle Too Small: The saddle is "perched" on the horse's back; it tends to pinch at the contact areas; it rolls right or left; a pad doesn't fit easily under it.

2. Saddle Too Wide at Front: Although you may seem to be achieving 100 percent contact, when a saddle is too wide it lies on the spine and the withers with little or no clearance.

3. Saddle Too Narrow at Front: This condition creates a loss of position and weight distribution, and the saddle usually seeks the wrong position. There is a great deal of pinching in the withers and shoulder area.

4. Bridging: This condition creates a "four-legged chair" weight distribution of the saddle on the horse's back. Contact is lost in the middle, although level and position seemingly is there. There may be excessive movement of the saddle with a rider on board.

5. High Centering: This condition creates a concentrated area of pressure under the seat of the saddle, leaving

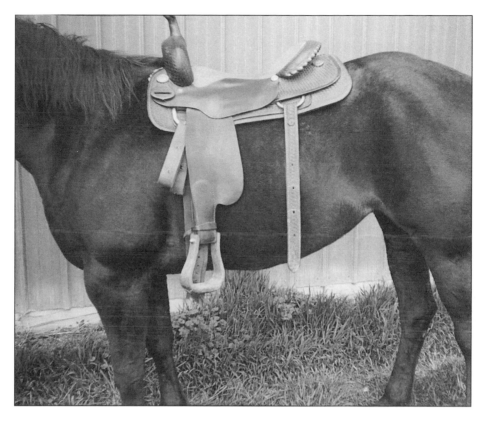

This saddle is clearly too wide, as it sits down on the horse's withers and spine, and too long, because it cuts into the horse's hip.

a fit that rocks front to back even when the girth is tight. This is also indicated by an uneven contact area.

6. Going Uphill and Downhill: A saddle tree has a manufactured level that dictates the function of the tree on horseback. Saddles that are not level show a downhill or uphill seat. By looking at a number of horses under saddle you can start to develop an eye for a level position (the lowest point of the seat). Attend workshops and work with your friends by placing different saddles on different horses and evaluating their fit.

Uphill seat to rider. The rider feels as though she is climbing to catch up with the motion. The saddle will tend to bring her leg too far under her as her seat continually slides back toward the cantle and she must constantly readjust to catch up. This is usually too

The same saddle shown on page 137 from a different view shows the lack of clearance at the withers and the pinching of the shoulders. It is too wide.

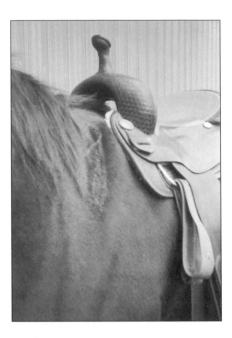

This English saddle causes pinching at the withers and has very little clearance for the spine. This, too, is a poor fit.

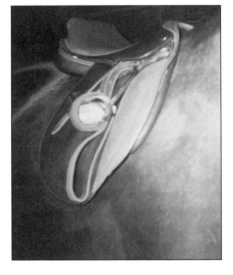

narrow a tree at the front. It will cause pressure to the loin area of the horse and generally create too much of a gap at the withers.

Downhill seat. Usually too wide a tree at the front causes this condition. As a consequence, a great deal of pressure is applied to the withers of the horse. Lack of contact and fishtailing at the cantle also result.

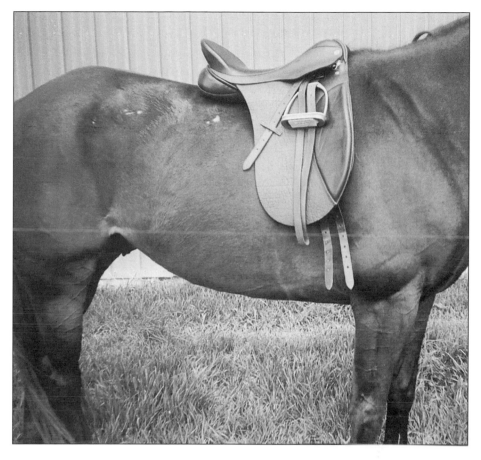

This saddle is set much too far forward and has an uphill seat. The rider's legs would keep moving forward and her seat would keep sliding backward.

Riders in these saddles will show an arched back position and feel as though they are riding on the forehand. The saddle may also cause them to want to shove their feet forward to stop themselves from sliding too far forward in the saddle toward the forehand.

7. Unhealthy Saddle Travel: When the saddle is not positioned correctly it will often travel or move to another fit position. This is unhealthy saddle travel—the saddle, affected by the conformation and motion of the horse, is trying to find a settled position. In so doing, it can injure the horse's back, often in more than one place

The rider who doesn't understand proper saddle fit may resort to cinches, breast straps, cruppers, and pads to remedy the situation. These quick fixes will maintain an incorrect saddle fit or position. When the saddle slips it is seeking a correct space. Beause it is not stable (or correctly fit), it moves. A correct fit will not move.

Here is an example of a downhill saddle on a downhill horse. Notice how the seat (the lowest point) tends to send your eye toward the horse's neck.

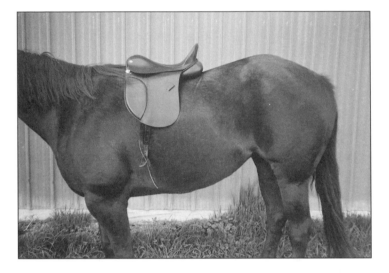

Here is a level saddle on the same downhill horse. You can see how this could make a tremendous amount of difference to rider and horse.

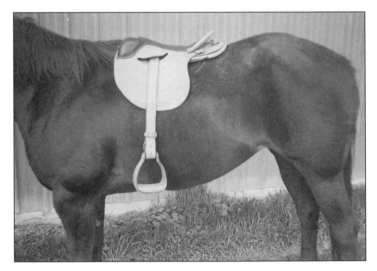

Steps to Proper Fit

1. Evaluate the horse to be saddled

   a. Visual inspection. Check:

   Symmetry of body

   Hooves and shoeing, mouth, general health and condition

   Obvious wounds to back, and treat

   Attitude of the horse

   b. Palpate:

   Check for deep wounds or soreness; note horse's reaction.

   Check horse's normal back posture every few months as the seasons, work and feed change.

   c. Inspect for fit:

   Horse stripped

   Horse with saddle and girth only

   Horse with pad, saddle and girth

   Horse with rider, pad, saddle and girth.

   - Evaluate from all sides and watch for behavior abnormalities with each stage.

   - Walk horse away from you and watch for overall back movement and one-sidedness; arching and lowering back (a horse on the bit will bring his back up, an unbalanced or nervous horse will go head high–hollow-backed) or in some cases, horses may go too deep (head to chest); and evenness of the side flexion or swing of the barrel as the horse turns in a serpentine.

2. Determine correct saddle fit.

   a. A saddle should center toward the natural seat position on the horse's back. This is usually the lowest point, over the fourteenth vertebrae.

This angle gives you an idea of how a good fit on the shoulder and withers looks. It is smooth and clear.

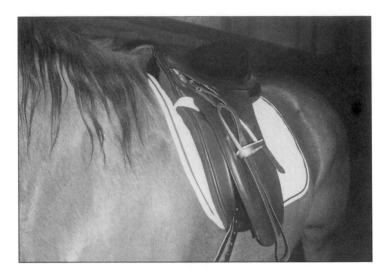

Another example of poor fit on a high-withered horse. The saddle should clear the withers and lie smoothly, as if molded on the horse's back.

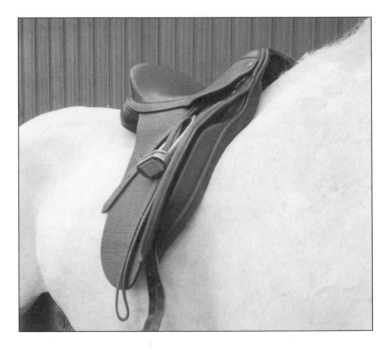

b. Saddles will move to the natural-fit position. It is here they must be fitted.

- Define margin of saddle contact area. Is there light showing through anywhere as you walk around the horse?

- *Withers area:* Hold four fingers together and place them stacked in between the withers and the pommel to assure clearance. With girth tightened you may drop to three fingers.

- *Shoulder area:* The saddle should not interfere with the shoulder. It must be positioned behind the rear of the scapula (shoulder). With a flat hand under the pommel, move down along the shoulder area.

Check out the margin of contact when you are inspecting a saddle. Notice that this saddle shows daylight under the seat area and is guilty of bridging. Photo: Rich Frasier.

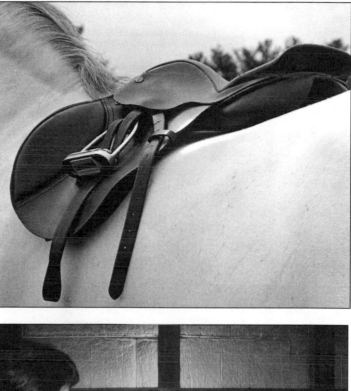

To check for clearance of the withers, place four fingers under the pommel without the girth tightened and then three fingers with the girth tightened.

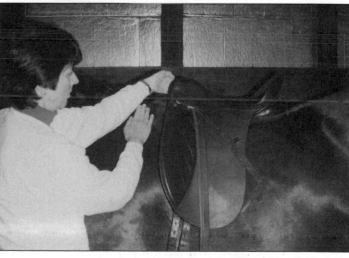

Make sure your saddle clears the shoulders by running your hand under the flaps with and without the girth tightened.

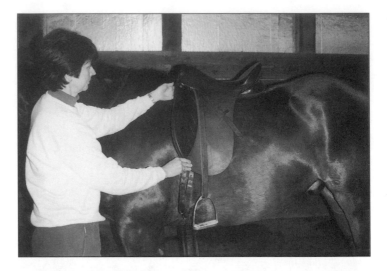

This saddle is obviously way too tight even to begin clearing the shoulder.

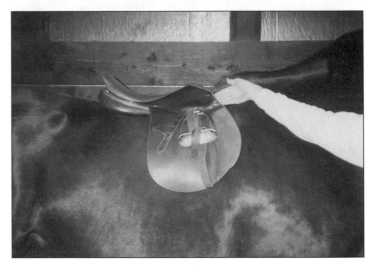

Is the saddle tight against the shoulder, or is there clearance for the shoulder to move naturally? If it is tight, try moving the saddle back first. If you still have difficulty clearing your hand under the front flap, your saddle is interfering with the shoulder's range of motion.

- *Loin area*: Do not contact rise of loin (point of hip) or loin area. Especially with western and endurance saddles, there must be at least four inches (or a flat hand's distance) between the back of the saddle and the point of hip.

This western saddle appears to fit but upon inspection, Peggy cannot even get her fingers in between the saddle and the withers.

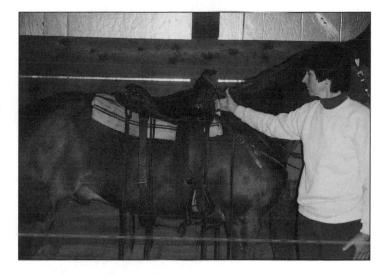

- *Spine:* Check from the rear that there is no contact with the spinous process (spinal area). The tree must stabilize on either side of the spine and never contact the spine.

c. Check for stability

- The saddle should not teeter or rock from front to back or side to side. It should be stable and level.

3. Shims and Pads. *Shims* are sections of "padding" used under your saddle to correct saddle fit. They can act as a wedge to fill a gap and make up the difference in a poor fit. But if done incorrectly they can add to the problem. In other words, talk to an expert. Some ill-fitting saddles can be corrected through shimming or redistribution. The saddle that is too small for the horse is the exception.

Saddle pads or blankets are used to keep the horse's back free of dirt and sweat (and to advertise sponsors). The ideal is to use a thin cotton or quilted pad and a saddle that fits correctly.

Some corrective pads can change the shape and size of the horse's back, which avoids, not remedies the problems.

Nonfunctional or straight padding simply adds another layer of poor fit. The ill fit has not been corrected by the padding.

A good way to tell if a saddle is too long and will interfere with the hindquarters is to see if there is a hand's width between the back of the saddle and the hips. If you can't fit your hand there, it is too long. Photo: Rich Frasier.

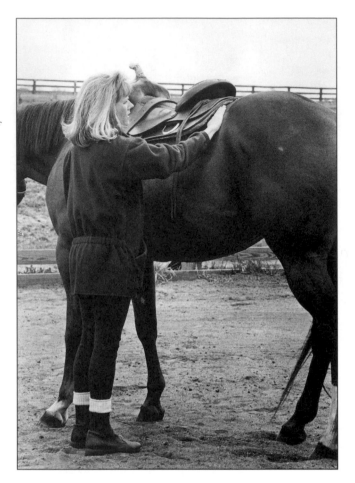

Functional padding. Padding that will mold, adjust to shape, and absorb shock—can help remedy a poor fit.

Always re-evaluate the entire saddle fit with each correction made. Often a problem doesn't become obvious until you are moving.

New or Custom Saddles

The final component of saddle fitting is to do it in the context of a new or custom fit saddle using the considerations and strategies just described.

Selecting a New Saddle

The ideal way to select a saddle is to load up the horse and ship him to the local tack store. This way, you won't be

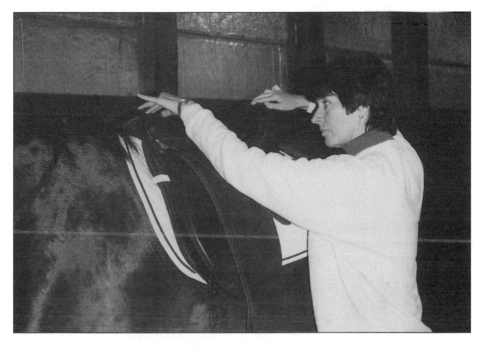

The saddle should not teeter or rock from front to back or side to side. It should be stable and solid.

Using a shim at the front and a pad levels the fit of this saddle.

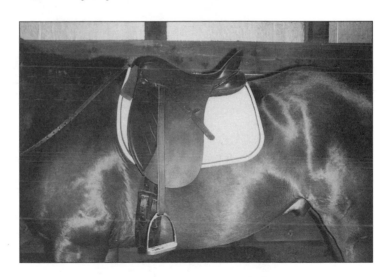

guessing and bringing a different saddle home every day to try it out. Have a professional saddle fitter meet you there to determine the best one for you and your horse.

Make sure the horse is clean and positioned in a secured parking lot or a safe area. Begin trying on various saddles (with and without a lightweight, thin pad).

A saddle such as this is too wide on this high-withered, low-backed horse.

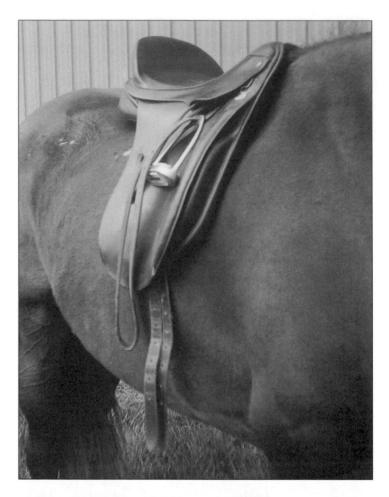

With the addition of a shim to lift and fill in the wither area, this saddle now fits much better, but it is still not perfect in the rear. The saddle is usable, however.

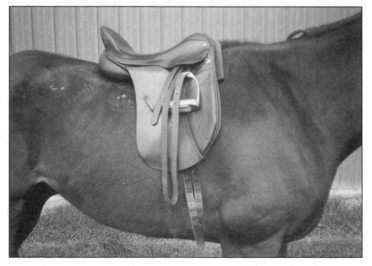

A great fit with no help: A clean, lightweight pad and a saddle that is level and clears the moving parts.

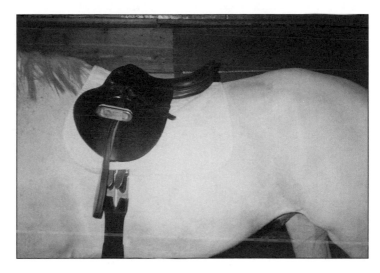

Extreme conditions such as high withers with a drastic dip down to the back or "mattress back" (a flat, wide back with little or no withers) are the most difficult to fit successfully. You may have to consider a custom saddle for horses with extreme conformation faults.

Custom Saddle

For custom fitting, you can have a professional come to your barn and measure your horse. The fitter will evaluate every aspect of your horse's size, breed, use, age and conformation, and should also take into account your plans and the environment in which the horse is being used. Your attributes such as age, experience and fitness should also be taken into consideration as well.

Recent Research in Women's Saddles

Paul Belton, chairman of Albion Saddlemakers Co., Ltd., of Walsall, England, and his associate, Dr. Sandra Dean, a physician and an experienced rider, recently joined forces to research and create a saddle for the female rider. There are several female-oriented saddles available in a growing market, but Albion has become a research and design leader in this area with its "comfort seat" for women, and plans to do much more.

Belton and Dean had unlimited use of libraries, skeletons and materials to research a prototype for the female rider. As Penny Goring noted in her article "Vive la

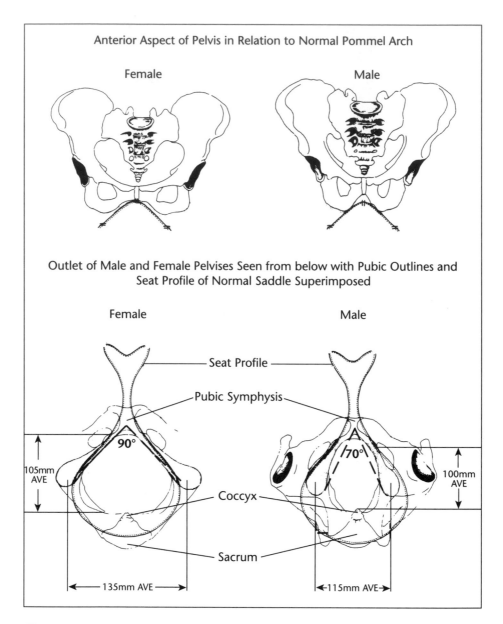

Anterior Aspect of Pelvis in Relation to Normal Pommel Arch

Female

Male

Outlet of Male and Female Pelvises Seen from below with Pubic Outlines and Seat Profile of Normal Saddle Superimposed

Female

Male

Seat Profile

Pubic Symphysis

90°

105mm AVE

70°

100mm AVE

Coccyx

Sacrum

135mm AVE

115mm AVE

The upper portion of this illustration shows the female pelvis and the male pelvis as if we were facing them. They are sitting in a saddle and their seat bones are placed on either side of the pommel. Notice the differences, especially contact with the saddle.

The lower portion of the illustration gives a view of the pelvises as if we were under them looking up through the saddle. Observe the differences in the placement and distribution of weight and balance. Information such as this about female anatomy is important to manufacturers and designers of saddles for women. Illustration: Courtesy of Jan Jacobson, Performance Saddlery.

Différénce?" (*Dressage*, 1988), "Placing the saddle underneath both male and female skeletons was a revelation and explained, by observation, why feel was bound to be different in the sexes. Although both sit on the ischial tuberosities, the natural tilt of the female pelvis places a woman's point of contact in front of the center of balance. This position is less stable, has a tendency to rock and the wider pubic arch is pushed forward onto the rigid arch of the pommel."

Belton and Dean had identified a basic positional difference that had direct consequences for the way women ride. What's more: "Studying the angle of the femur provided a further clue. In a classical gynaecoid pelvis, which 80 percent of women have, the seam line lies against the inner thigh, causing great discomfort. It is not only the bone structure that is different; the covering ligaments in the female stretch easily, making the whole pelvic girdle weaker and less well protected. The male pelvis, on the other hand, not only has a thick fleshy pad over the pubic arch, giving him extra protection, but the straighter angle of the femur keeps him well inside the seam line."

The varying shapes of the female pelvis explained why some women are comfortable in ordinary saddles: Their particular shape just happened to fit the saddle. But the larger conclusion was obvious: Female riders are different, and have different saddle requirements.

The design process that followed produced a saddle that was better able to offer a secure and pain-free ride and that allowed the female rider to use her weight more effectively. According to Goring, "(Trot) Extensions in particular have been markedly improved, since the lady rider no longer has to change her position to protect herself."

Chapter 8

Fuel Up for High-Energy Performance

with Margaret (Peg) M. McGovern

A "fit" body needs a healthful diet to fuel physical performance.
—Sarah C. Parks, Past President of the American Dietetic
Association

We live in a time when knowledge about food and its relationship to health and fitness is advancing rapidly. As riders we understand that what goes into our horses matters, so it doesn't require too much additional insight to recognize that what goes into *us* matters too. If you want to be treated like an athlete (and achieve like an athlete), you have to behave like one. That doesn't mean endless sacrifice, although some degree certainly is necessary. It does mean cultivating a sense of responsibility to the ultimate goal of good performance. And that means eating right.

To fill the gap between our needs and our awareness, I initiated a search for a sports nutrition specialist who was interested in relating experience in that field to the world of the rider, specifically the female rider. Enter Margaret (Peg) M. McGovern, M.B.A., a licensed and registered dietitian who was the assistant director of Food and Nutrition Services at the Georgetown University Medical Center in Washington, D.C. for over ten years. I've taught Peg a great deal about horse sports, and she has taught me a great deal about how to fuel riders' bodies for their activities with horses.

What follows is the result of our collaboration on nutrition and the female rider.

Peg's initial observations tracked with mine: The area of nutrition for female equestrians has not been addressed or researched in comparison with other sport and recreational activities. And she immediately realized that equestrian sports have very different demands from other sports. Even those who ride occasionally at an easy pace need to know how to prepare their body to ride. By preparing your body nutritionally you will enjoy riding more, feel less fatigue, have more endurance and attain better balance and movement with your horse. Ultimately, you will see your physical well-being reflected in the horse's performance.

The female equestrian's preparation to ride includes hours of feeding, grooming and exercising her horse. She feeds her horse a balanced, high-quality diet and supplements for maximum conditioning. She provides clean water for proper hydration, and gives her horse sufficient exercise to maintain muscle tone and mental health. The horse has been properly fueled and exercised for performance. So what about the other half of the team? The long hours spent before and after the ride and riding itself can take a toll on the pilot. Too often, she stops just long enough to snack on what's quick to pack, inexpensive, available, easy to carry and nonperishable. Many women say there's never enough time to eat right when working with horses.

AWAREness

If you're paying more attention to what your horse eats than to what you eat, you have some rethinking to do.

If you think about how important you are to your horse's health and how much you affect his well-being and performance, you'll reach a different conclusion. Female riders need to uphold their 50 percent of the intake bargain. Your personal nutrition is the key to feeling well and performing at your best.

Knowledge of the physical demands of your horse activities, exercise and proper rest will enhance your own performance. Now let's add good nutrition to the list of things we know how to handle. The question is how to fuel the body for maximum appearance and performance. As with your horse, the combination of certain foods provides a balance of nutrients such as carbohydrates, proteins, fats and essential vitamins and minerals. The key is to eat foods that fuel the body appropriately and provide sufficient energy for your needs.

Below, we discuss what your system needs and offer some recommendations. The "Food Guide Pyramid,"(see page 167) published by the U.S. Department of Health and Human Services, is used to identify carbohydrate, protein and fat in foods that deliver energy to the body as calories. "Dietary Guidelines for Americans," developed by the U.S. Department of Agriculture and the U.S. Department of Health and Human Services, are used to plan a healthy diet before, during and after competitions.

Just as we did with our exercise program, we are laying out the possibilities for you. Depending on your personal objectives and limitations (if any), you may choose to pursue some of the recommendations and disregard others. You decide. Our goal is to make sure you know what the options are.

Body Fuel: Carbohydrates, Protein and Fat

The *carbohydrate* is the only *ergogenic* aid known to satisfy energy needs and produce desired results. Ergogenic foods are nutritional substances which are believed to support or stimulate the athletic performance. Carbohydrates should comprise approximately 55 to 65 percent of our daily food intake. Complex carbohydrates, the preferred anaerobic food, should be emphasized because they increase glycogen, which stores more efficiently than simple carbohydrates and provides the high-energy source for peak performance. Starches such as breads, whole grains, cereals, pasta and legumes are excellent sources of complex carbohydrates. Try to include six to eleven servings in your diet each day. Simple carbohydrates, which provide quick energy, are found in fruits and vegetables. Include two to four servings of fruits and three to five servings of vegetables in your diet each day. All of these food groups provide necessary electrolytes, vitamins and minerals. Fortunately these foods, which can be included in the weekly grocery trip, are quick to fix, easy to carry and store, and taste good.

Carbohydrate Strategy

1. Create a snack mix high in carbohydrates and low in fat by using your favorite cereal mix. At the end of this section, you'll find my favorite recipe, which you

might want to modify to suit yourself—or make up your own recipe. Possible components include toasted bagel chips, pretzels, low-fat snack crackers, vanilla wafers, gingersnaps, low-fat granola, plain or flavored rice cakes, flavored bread sticks, air-popped popcorn (with your preferred seasoning such as salt, imitation butter or cheese flavoring, cinnamon, nutmeg or hot spices). Add a favorite dry cereal if you wish.

2. Make enough snack mix for the week. Carry plastic bags with your favorite mixes in the glove compartment of your car.

3. Raw vegetables like celery and carrot sticks don't have the same shelf life (and don't qualify for extended glove compartment storage) but nonetheless are easy to keep on hand. The rider who eats a raw carrot meets her requirements for vitamin A for the day. Fresh and dried fruit like apples, grapes, pears, bananas and raisins are easy to store and travel well in all kinds of weather.

4. Like Mom said, sharing is good, so don't forget to offer a few of those apples and carrots to your horse. The motive here is a little selfish. If you get in the habit of having an apple or carrot break with your horse, you can cut down on your own craving for some of those "empty calorie" people foods.

Protein is the structural component of all body tissues necessary for growth and repair. Proteins should comprise approximately 15 to 18 percent of daily food intake. The average protein intake *per serving* is approximately 3 ounces, which translates into 21 grams of protein or 165 calories. The typical female equestrian requires the average Recommended Daily Allowance of .8 grams/kg body weight, or two to three servings. If she is active in strength and endurance athletics, she may need as much as 1 to 1.5 grams/kg body weight. In general, we tend to eat far more protein than our bodies need or can use.[1] *If the female rider is eating a balanced diet, she will not need to eat additional protein.* Excellent sources of protein include fish, chicken, turkey, lean

---

[1] It is important, while we are discussing protein, to note that recent research shows that protein and amino acid supplements are expensive and ineffective in promoting endurance and/or increasing muscle mass.

pork and beef. Other sources of high-quality protein are lentils, nuts and dairy products.

Protein Strategy

1. Substitute chicken, turkey or fish for traditional beef, hamburger, meat loaf, pork, bacon and sausage entrees to achieve protein needs with decreased saturated fat, lower cholesterol content and fewer calories.

2. Lower calorie intake even further by baking, broiling, grilling, steaming or boiling your meat or fish entrees.

3. For the vegetarian, choose low-fat veggie burgers, tofu, legumes, lentils, nuts and dairy products.

4. When stopping at a convenience store for a quick, cheap snack, grab a package of string cheese made from skim milk, or a low-fat yogurt. For extra crunchiness, mix your favorite cereal or our recommended snack into the yogurt.

Fat is the third energy source for fueling the body. Fat supplies the body with essential fatty acids required for growth and maintenance of skin integrity. It provides and carries important fat-soluble vitamins such as A, D, E and K. But as we all know, fat has consequences that make us pay attention to how much of it is going into our bodies. Calories from fat should comprise no more than 20 to 25 percent of daily food intake.

Fat requirements for the equestrian female are the same as for all females. The overall reason is also pretty much the same: Lower fat intake in our diet helps reduce risk factors for heart disease, cancer and obesity.

Two types of fat in the diet are saturated and unsaturated fat. Sometimes fats are referred to as being "good fat" (mono- or polyunsaturated) or "bad fat" (saturated, which increases blood cholesterol). Monounsaturated and polyunsaturated fats may be defined chemically as fatty acids that contain single and double bonds, respectively. Olive oil is a source of monounsaturated fat; other vegetable and salad oils such as corn, sunflower, safflower and cottonseed oil are sources of polyunsaturated fats. Saturated fat may be defined chemically as fatty acids with many hydrogen bonds attached to the carbon and oxygen bonds. The more hydrogen, the higher the saturation, which simplistically can be pictured as "heavy" and hence, not particularly good for you. Saturated fats are found in marbled meats, poultry skin and hydrogenated (hard) fats such as butter or lard.

As annoying as it may seem, we need to monitor or count the fat grams in our diet. *What really counts is the percentage of total calories from fat sources.* One gram of fat contains nine calories, and it takes longer to burn than carbohydrates and protein. One gram of carbohydrate or protein, by comparison, contains only four calories.

Fat Strategy

1. Fat consciousness may be "trendy," but it's a trend that's almost certainly here to stay. Use food labels to check the fat content of food items, and remember to check for the portion size.

2. When preparing foods, purchase lean cuts of meat, skin poultry whenever practical and trim visible fat as much as possible. Use a non-stick pan or vegetable spray. Use low-fat or fat-free salad dressing and low-fat or fat-free dairy products.

3. When eating out, be sure to ask for salad dressing on the side. Entrees, vegetables and starches may be ordered without butter, margarine, sour cream or cream sauces. (I've found plain yogurt with some seasoning to be as satisfying as sour cream.)

4. If you must use margarine, do so at the table where you can control the amount used, as opposed to using it in the cooking process. Remember, a small variance in fat intake in the diet for one meal (25 to 60 grams) can make a big difference over time.

5. Pay attention to news concerning guidelines on reducing fat in the diet, particularly that coming from the American Heart Association, the National Research Council and the U.S. Department of Agriculture.

Your horse will appreciate your attention to fat. In addition to the most obvious reason—less weight on you means less weight on the horse—there are direct implications for your ability to effect a good, secure seat and feel the response of the horse in key parts of your body. If you're carrying too much extra weight, you won't have as much stamina in the saddle as the fit rider.

It's not a crime to satisfy your sweet tooth with cookies and cake snacks. Just try to monitor the portion size and number of servings, and make an effort to find a lower-fat product you like. Peg defines "low fat" as less than three grams of fat per serving, and there are many fine products to select from in the low-fat and fat-free categories.

AWAREness

If you have been doing so, stop writing off fat-reduced products as unacceptable and get with the program of experimenting to find the ones you like best.

If a quick fix of energy is needed, there are many "high calorie, high nutrient" drinks, cookies and bars available in food, drug and sports stores. These products will provide additional calories and a source of energy in a condensed, easy-to-carry form.

Any sensible, well-balanced diet will provide the female rider with adequate amounts of vitamins and minerals. Keep in mind that vitamins and minerals do not supply energy. If a female rider senses that she needs an additional supplement in her diet, such as the mineral calcium, she should seek the advice of a reputable professional—her doctor or a registered or licensed dietitian.

Based on the information we are providing in this chapter, you may want to consult a professional dietitian and design a plan to meet your lifestyle and horse-related activities.

Anyone may contact the American Dietetic Association through the direct consumer line at 1-800-366-1655 to inquire about local nutrition associations or private nutrition consultants. Fees for consultations range from forty to seventy-five dollars per hour, depending on area of the country and client needs.

Fluids: A Key to Riding

Fluid intake and replacement is crucial to the health and safety of the female rider, especially during warm weather and events on hot days. Just like nutrition in general, here's another area in which we expend a great deal of time, effort and worry over the proper treatment of our horses, (access to fluids, electrolyte supplements, etc.) and seem to forget about our own. Water in the body maintains normal body temperature and acts as a coolant for working muscles. When the body is warmer than the air around it, we begin to sweat in order to effect the necessary heat loss. In general, water and cool fluids regulate the body temperature, ease the pressure on joints and are essential to keeping a cool head when mounted during especially stressful situations. This puts a premium on maintaining necessary fluid levels during extended exertions with our horses.

Riding comes with a particular set of circumstances that are cause for concern. Currently show rules require equestrians to wear tight-fitting outfits such as jeans and chaps, dark-colored jackets, high collars and long-sleeved shirts, black heavy helmets or Stetsons and leather boots with no ventilation. Most of this clothing only adds warmth and in many cases increases the internal body temperature to dangerous levels. This leads to excess perspiration, creating the possibility of dehydration, disorientation, misjudgment and dizziness. Female riders in such circumstances especially need to take in fluids (hydrate) often.

Water is the best choice for replacement of body fluids. Female riders require an average of eight to ten cups of water each day, plus an additional two to four cups if the environment, type of performance, heat and amount of elapsed time for the activity combine to create the need. A dark urine color after competition, and for that matter anytime, indicates that you need to increase your intake of water.

AWAREness
Keep bottled water with you as much as possible. Keep several bottles at home and in the office, one always in your car or truck and at the barn. Consider bottled water especially when you are traveling. Your body may not adjust well to "foreign" water and you need your body working for you when nerves are high at competitions.

Fluids Strategy

1. Drink plenty of fluids throughout the day, and don't try to lose weight by cutting down on fluids.

2. Concentrate on extra fluid intake prior to a competition or extended work period. Don't wait until afterwards when you have an unquenchable thirst and/or a headache—both are signs of dehydration. Some beverages that may be substituted for water include juices, flavored bottled waters and even milk.

3. Avoid or reduce beverages containing caffeine and food containing chocolate (which contains caffeine). Beverages containing alcohol and those containing caffeine (such as coffee, tea and cola) act as diuretics, which cause you to lose water through increased urination.

4. The female facing premenstrual fluid retention may want to be careful about fluids and foods included in the diet. Avoid high-salt or -sodium beverages and foods such as vegetable juices and snack chips because sodium in those foods increases fluid retention.

Ideal Body Weight and Caloric Intake for the Female Rider

Sorry, but your horse wants you to know about weight and calories!

Ideal body weight is normally defined and determined by the 1983 Metropolitan Height-Weight Tables published by the Metropolitan Life Insurance Company. These tables give ideal average weights according to sex, height and frame size. While not absolute, these tables indicate roughly where you should be.

Metlife Female Height and Weight Table[1]

Height	Small Frame	Medium Frame	Large Frame
4'10"	102–111	109–121	118–131
4'11"	103–113	111–123	120–134
5'	104–115	113–126	122–137
5'1"	106–118	115–129	125–140
5'2"	108–121	118–132	128–143
5'3"	111–124	121–135	131–147
5'4"	114–127	124–138	134–151
5'5"	117–130	127–141	137–155
5'6"	120–133	130–144	140–159

[1] Weights at ages 25–29 based on lowest mortality. Weight in pounds according to frame, including clothing weighing 3 pounds.

Metlife Female Height and Weight Table (cont.)

Height	Small Frame	Medium Frame	Large Frame
5'7"	123–136	133–147	143–163
5'8"	126–139	136–150	146–167
5'9"	129–142	139–153	149–170
5'10"	132–145	142–156	152–173
5'11"	135–148	145–159	155–176
6'	138–151	148–162	158–179

To approximate your frame size, bend your forearm upward at a 90-degree angle. Keep fingers straight and turn the inside of your wrist toward your body. Place thumb and index finger of other hand on the two prominent bones on either side of the elbow. Measure space between your fingers on a ruler. Compare with the tables below listing elbow measurements for medium-framed women.

Female Elbow Measurements to Determine Medium Frame

Height in 1" Heels	Elbow Breadth
4'10"–4'11"	$2\frac{1}{4}$" to $2\frac{1}{2}$"
5'–5'3"	$2\frac{1}{4}$" to $2\frac{1}{2}$"
5'4"–5'7"	$2\frac{3}{8}$" to $2\frac{5}{8}$"
5'8"–5'11"	$2\frac{3}{8}$" to $2\frac{5}{8}$"
6'+	$2\frac{1}{2}$" to $2\frac{3}{4}$"

Measurements lower than those listed indicate a small frame. Higher measurements indicate a large frame.

Also, here's a simple calculation (called the Hamwi Formula) that can be used to help calculate your ideal body weight.

- Start with 100 pounds for the first five feet.

- Add five pounds for each inch of your height over five feet.

You may adjust total average weight by 10 percent depending on your body frame. If your body frame is small, decrease your average weight; if your body frame is large, add to your average weight.

Female Medium Frame

Height	5'4"	5'7"
First 5'	100	100
Additional inches at five pounds each	20 (4 × 5)	35 (7 × 5)
Total Ideal Weight	120	135

Your ideal weight establishes a target that can be pursued by modifying your diet and understanding the calorie expenditures associated with your horse activities.

Many factors must be considered when calculating calorie requirements. For example, the female equestrian's metabolic rate and calorie expenditures are greatly influenced by her age, body size and basal metabolism, in addition to type of activity, duration, frequency and intensity of training and performance. The basal metabolism is the total energy used by the body at rest for breathing, cell growth and repair.

The rider's energy needs are determined by her basal metabolic requirement, food intake, digestion and physical activity. The body produces energy from the carbohydrate, protein and fat that we eat after the foods have been digested and metabolized for use as energy in the form of glycogen and glucose.

The Harris Benedict equation is commonly used to calculate calorie requirements. Using it, we can calculate calorie expenditures for twenty-four hours based on sex, age and size. The activity factor code provides the approximate energy expenditure for the level of activity, whether the activity is sedentary, somewhat active or very active. Average activity factor codes are listed below. Using the examples, an equestrian can calculate daily energy/calorie requirements using the following activity codes and formula. (A kilogram [kg] is a metric unit of weight. One pound of body weight is equal to 2.2 kilograms of body weight in the metric system. Body weight formula for conversion of pounds to kilograms: Pounds ÷ 2.2 = kilograms body weight.)

Element 1: Basic Calorie Needs
Your basic calorie intake level is determined by your classification based on activity:

Activity Factor Code

20 = adult /sedentary; desk job; no routine exercise

25 = adult/active; walking on the job; some exercise

40 = adolescent/active; regular exercise

Multiplying this code by your weight gives you a total base calorie intake per day. For a 120-pound, moderately active female:

1. 120 pounds ÷ 2.2 kilograms body weight = 54.5 Kg body weight

2. 54.5 kilograms × 25 (active adult) = 1,363 calories/day

So, if you are 5'4" and medium frame (as in the earlier example), your ideal weight is 120. If you are above that, you can pursue the target either by taking in fewer calories, burning more, or some combination of the two. Now let's take a look at how horse activities fit in.

Element 2: Energy Expenditures
Peg McGovern and her associates determined that horse-related activities burn calories at the following rates:

Calories Burned per Minute of Activity

Horse-grooming = 0.128

Galloping = 0.137

Trotting = 0.110

Walking = 0.041

Using these rates, we can determine calorie burn totals for the days on which you work with your horse(s).

For example, for a 120-pound female *grooming* a horse:

1. 0.128 (kcal/min) × 54.5 Kg/body weight)
   = **6.9 cal/min**

2. 30 minutes spent grooming × 6.9 cal/min
   = **207 calories**

In other words, horse grooming expends 6.9 calories per minute for this woman, and thirty minutes of it burns more than 200 calories.

You can calculate the total for all of your horse activities by using the chart below and filling in (1) your body weight (in kilograms) and (2) the number of minutes you spend on the activity in question:

Activity	Kcal/ Minute	×	Rider body weight (kg)	×	Minutes	=	Total Expended Calories
Horse-grooming	0.128	×		×		=	
Galloping	0.137	×		×		=	
Trotting	0.110	×		×		=	
Walking	0.041	×		×		=	
Total							

A day which included thirty minutes of grooming, twenty minutes of galloping, thirty minutes of trotting and ten minutes of walking would produce the following calorie profile:

Equestrian Activity	=	Calories/min	×	min.	=	Calorie Expenditure
Horse grooming	=	6.9	×	30	=	207 calories
Galloping	=	7.4	×	20	=	148 calories
Trotting	=	5.9	×	30	=	177 calories
Walking	=	2.2	×	10	=	22 calories
Total						**554 calories**

There is no research data available which differentiates between females and males doing these energy-expending sports.

Let's compare our sport to other activities. A 5'4" to 5'5", 143-pound woman expends the following calories per minute in these activities.[2]

[2] W.D. McArdle, et al. *Exercise Physiology,* 3rd ed.

Calories Expended per Minute of Activity

Sport	Calories Expended
Backstroke swimming (laps)	11.0
Cross-country running	10.6
Galloping	**7.4**
Tennis	7.1
Horse-grooming	**6.9**
Medium- to low-impact aerobics	6.7
Snow skiing	6.4
Trotting	**5.9**
Walking	5.2
Sweeping the floor	2.9
Walking (on horseback)	**2.2**

As you can see, equestrian activities are right up there with high-energy activities. We burn a great deal in preparation to ride.

Weight Loss Through Management, Not Diets

Using the above, you can figure out where you are and what you have to do in order to move toward your ideal or target weight. Simply put, diet management and exercise are the only safe means to that end.

Recent research has indicated that "yo-yo" dieting and poor nutrition affect metabolism by making it difficult to adjust to the desired basal metabolic rate for weight maintenance and energy requirement during physical activity or competition. Yo-yo dieting or binge dieting works in reverse of the desired effect. When you don't eat, your body acts to protect you from starvation. Your metabolism drops and your body produces more fat and sugar to take care of the deficit.

Diet Guidelines: Before and After a Competition

Some of us ride daily, while others ride and perform less frequently. Whether you compete regularly or just once in a while, the following basic guidelines should be followed.

1. Eat a balanced diet using the Food Guide Pyramid recommendations for adequate food energy (see below).

2. Follow the carbohydrate, protein and fat strategies described earlier.

3. On the day of the horse show, plan to eat three to four hours prior to the event to allow adequate time for digestion.

4. Select a precompetition meal that is light and easy to digest—one possibility is described at the end of this section. Prior to an event, eat foods high in complex carbohydrates and moderate in protein. Avoid foods high in fat because they digest and absorb slowly.

5. Eat foods familiar to you and avoid foods that may cause gastric discomfort. You're going to be jostling around in the saddle and running around for hours under stress. The last thing you need is a heavy feeling or crampy stomach. Foods that digest slowly and can cause discomfort include cabbage, onions and spicy and fried foods.

The Food Guide Pyramid

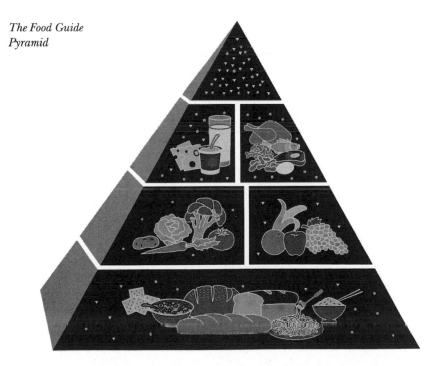

6. After the event, rehydrate with fluid. Water is the fluid of choice, followed by juices and beverages without caffeine. Get in the habit of carrying bottled water with you wherever you go.

Night-Before Meal

Many athletes choose pasta for a precompetition dinner (the night before). One of our favorites is offered below. This dinner contains 1,081 calories—66 percent carbohydrate, 12 percent protein, 22 percent fat.

Menu

Beverage   6 oz. Cranberry Juice Spritzer

Rigatoni with Italian Tomato Sauce

2 cups rigatoni or spaghetti

1 cup Italian spaghetti sauce with your favorite spices (recipe below)

1 large tossed green salad

2 tbsp. low-fat Italian dressing (on the side)

2 slices Italian bread

2 tsp. margarine

If meat sauce is desired, add 1 or 2 ounces sautéed lean ground turkey breast and season to taste.

Recipe for Meatless Sauce

Makes 8–10 servings (Freezes well for a show season—about 3 months)

1 24 oz. can tomato sauce

3 6 oz. cans tomato paste

3 28 oz. cans cooking tomatoes

1 tsp. sugar (optional)

2 oz. grated Parmesan cheese

2 tbsp. seasonings (Italian oregano, thyme, etc.)

3 garlic cloves—minced

2 tbsp. dry parsley or 1/4 cup fresh parsley

4 oz. water

salt and pepper to taste

Step 1: Puree cooking tomatoes in blender. Put all ingredients (unless you prefer a sauce with meat—read step 2) in a large heavy pot.

Step 2: For a sauce with meat: In a nonstick pan, sauté 1 lb. of ground turkey with the crushed garlic cloves, parsley, Parmesan cheese, salt and pepper. Drain fat drippings and add meat mixture to tomato sauce and remaining ingredients.

Simmer for four to six hours over low heat. The longer the sauce simmers, the better.

Suggestions: Cook sauce two to three hours, refrigerate overnight and continue cooking the next day. Add vegetables or mushrooms for variety a few minutes before serving.

Step 3: Cook rigatoni or spaghetti according to package directions. Spoon sauce over pasta and sprinkle with Parmesan cheese if you prefer.
Freeze in individual containers for later use.

No time to prepare and wait for sauce to cook? Purchase one of the many kinds of commercially prepared sauces. Remember to read the food label for fat content, which can vary considerably from product to product.

Breakfast Options

Breakfast is very important for the rider. Even though many riders say they are too nervous to eat, your body needs the nutrition to help cope with stress and exertion. It will take two or three hours for the following breakfast to be digested and you will have fueled your body for the morning's competition.

Light Breakfast for an Early-Morning Competition (6:30 AM meal)

764 calories: 83 percent carbohydrate, 12 percent protein, 5 percent fat

8 oz. apple juice

1 fresh orange

1 or 2 whole wheat bagels or toast

2 tbsp. honey or jam

8 oz. skim milk

Breakfast for an Afternoon Competition (Later morning meal)

936 calories:
73 percent carbo-
hydrate, 10 per-
cent protein,
17 percent fat

1/2 banana

4 oz. grape juice

2 slices whole grain toast

2 oz. dry cereal

2 tbsp. jelly

2 tsp. margarine

8 oz. skim milk

Water

Pack your breakfast the night before if you're traveling in the early morning hours.

All of these items can be eaten in the car. Place juice and milk in a small cooler or enjoy these beverages before you leave home.

Snacking

As mentioned earlier, keeping wholesome snacks with you is important for maintaining your energy level and avoiding the urge to pick up junk food along the way.

The **AWARE** *Snack—Quick Nutty Cereal Mix*

A. 2 cups Rice Krispies

2 cups Bran Chex

2 cups Wheat or Corn Chex

3 cups Cheerios

1 cup unsalted dry-roasted peanuts

1 cup golden raisins

1 8 oz. pkg. Indian Hot Mix (optional)

B. 2 tbsp. olive oil

1 1/2 tsp. cumin seed

chili powder to taste

1/2 tsp. turmeric powder

1/4 tsp. garlic powder

1/2 tsp. sugar

1 Tbsp. dry parsley

salt to taste

Step 1. Gently mix all the ingredients in Step A.

Step 2. In Step B, put oil in saucepan over medium heat. Lower the heat and add cumin seeds, followed by turmeric powder, chili powder and garlic powder. Stir and add to cereal mix. Add nuts, raisins, salt, sugar and dried parsley. Toss gently. Store in airtight container.

Step 3. Be creative and use your favorite cereal, pretzel sticks, coconut and dried fruits.

Step 4. Place in individual plastic bags for quick snacks in the car or at the barn.

Tips for Eating away from Home

Eating Out

- Select broiled or grilled burger. Don't order deep-fat–fried entrees.

- Select lean meat, seafood or mixed green salads with dressing on the side.

- Select a baked potato without the butter, sour cream, cheese and bacon. If you have to use condiments, order them on the side and use sparingly.

- For breakfast, order dry cereal with fruit and skim milk. Avoid "traditional" heavy orders such as bacon and eggs with hash browns.

- Carry your own fruit. Avoid high-fat, rich desserts. (If you have to splurge every now and then, order one serving for the table with several forks or spoons.)

- Order decaffeinated beverages.

Driving in the Car or Van

- Pack your breakfast and light low-fat snacks.

- Keep fresh or dried fruits available.

- Keep low-fat crackers or cookies on hand.

- For bread on sandwiches or as a snack, use bagels or Melba toast.

- Always include juice or bottled water.

Chapter 9

Growth, Pregnancy and Aging

Mature and married women can ride side-saddle with impunity often to a great age, but whether they can do so astride is a matter for the medical profession to decide.—Lt. Col. S. G. Goldschmidt, *The Fellowship of the Horse,* 1930

Women go through numerous physical, emotional and lifestyle changes throughout their lives. These changes affect how the female adapts to training, physiologically and biomechanically. Understanding and accepting these changes will not only enhance the enjoyment of riding but will also improve effectiveness and prevent injury.

Physical considerations such as bone growth and deterioration, flexibility or the lack thereof in the joints, hormonal changes and mood swings, skin and body hydration are key to the well-being and athletic success of the female rider throughout her life. At the same time, lifestyle, mental, emotional and spiritual issues play an equally important role.

Again with the help of Mary Beth Walsh, let's take a brief look at some of the phases of female development and how they relate to riding.

The Child Rider (Ages Six to Twelve)

During the childhood years, the female body undergoes very rapid growth. Growth spurts may affect flexibility. For example, it is not uncommon for a ten- or eleven-year-old girl to lose the ability to bend over and touch her toes, because her long bones are growing faster than her muscles.

The development of the spine is crucial in the prepubescent years (eleven to twelve). Scoliosis (spine curvature) is far more common in females than in males; the accelerated growth of the skeletal system is partly the cause. Signs of significant scoliosis should be referred to a doctor.

Riding is an excellent way to reinforce good posture and to strengthen postural muscles at a young age; in some cases, it is used as a therapeutic exercise. If used correctly, riding can benefit a girl physically and help her in other ways with the challenges growth presents.

The female body matures earlier than that of the male, a fact that becomes most noticeable around the age of eleven or twelve. It is not unusual that a female begins to master physical skills and is well-coordinated at this age. Although young riders have the physical ability and energy, they may not yet have developed a healthy appreciation of the injuries that might occur, which is why some extra guidance is desirable.

The Adolescent Rider (Ages Twelve to Eighteen)

The adolescent years are fraught with many problems, both physical and emotional. Biomechanically, a girl's body begins to assume a more feminine shape, compared to the more androgynous form of earlier years. The development of breasts and the increase in soft tissue around the hips alters the balance of a rider. She should be made aware that as these changes occur they may affect her riding.

This is an issue of rebalancing and not taking too much for granted on horseback—two themes to be mindful of always.

Certainly the changes of adolescence affect how a young woman may carry herself. Young women who are not yet comfortable with their new figure attempt to hide it by rounding their shoulders and slouching. Good posture is vital to overall health and for preventing damage to the back, as well as riding comfort. Self-esteem and balanced equitation go hand in hand as a young woman becomes more comfortable with her body and riding skills.

Of greater significance, as in the prepubescent years, is the increased incidence of scoliosis in females, which (along with the change in body composition) must be addressed

both on and off the saddle in the interest of musculoskeletal development and good postural habits.

Along with the biomechanical changes in her body, the
adolescent girl is also dealing with the onset of menses.
Cramping and water retention often affect the desire to
ride, but many experts contend that physical exercise, particularly something a girl enjoys, can help alleviate or minimize the symptoms.

At this age, it is difficult but nonetheless important for
a rider to inform her instructor if she does not feel up to
riding or participating in a strenuous training session. Conversely, riding instructors need to be sensitive to girls' needs
in the adolescent years. During certain phases of the menstrual cycle, some teens say they have more joint pain which
affects their riding. As we discussed earlier, this is due to
the hormone estrogen. An increase in estrogen causes a
decrease in the threshold for pain, particularly in the joints.
Awareness of your cycle and preparation through exercises,
nutrition and proper support undergarments, are especially
vital to minimize pain and maximize performance for young
and adult females participating in high impact sports such
as riding.

Many girls move from ponies to horses in a matter of
months during the time they are experiencing a tremendous growth spurt. "I had no idea how to handle my body
or the horse," one of them told me. "Mov-
ing from ponies to a horse was a very different feeling and no one talked about the
changes or acknowledged anything new that
was happening to me. It would have helped
a lot if my instructors had worked with me
through those growing years instead of continuing as though nothing had changed."

AWAREness

*Most injuries that occur during
adolescence are due to the
carelessness and unnecessary
risk-taking we typically associate
with youth. Most of these
injuries are preventable; luckily,
during this phase of life, the
female rider also heals quickly.*

Girls also should be paying attention to
and taking care of their skin at this age, especially because of the harsh nature of our
outdoor sporting environment. Skin cancer
begins with childhood sunburns. Young girls
spend many hours exposed to the elements,
particularly at summertime horse shows. Mothers and
friends need to encourage young female riders to protect

their skin from wind, sun and dirt with a good cleansing, moisturizing and protection program. A moisturizer with a minimum SPF of 15 should be used on the face and neck. The long-term consequences of not doing so are significant.

A girl of this age needs to be educated about her body so she understands how it affects her riding and her well-being. And she needs a good bit of understanding from us.

The Twenties and Thirties

At this phase of life, a rider generally enjoys being at the peak of her physical ability. However, young women often begin to feel the pressures of adult life encroaching on time spent at the stable and on maintaining fitness. This is the time of life that a solid fitness routine becomes a priority alongside going to work and paying the bills.

Riding alone does not provide the fitness required for performance, especially if you only ride occasionally. Like any other sport, riding requires that other athletic activities be added to the mix.

AWAREness

Most of the injuries that occur during this time of life are linked with the "Weekend Warrior" syndrome in which one suffers strains and sprains by attempting to perform at a previous level without the fitness to support the effort.

Because we have more demands made on our time during these years, we are less likely to maintain the level of fitness necessary to keep in shape to ride. The solution lies in a more consistent program of exercise throughout the week. Chapter 6 offers an exercise program that you can fit into a busy day of work and family along with caring for your horse.

At this age, women may want to become knowledgeable about pregnancy and riding (see page 180) and discuss it with their doctor. You should also be aware of hormonal changes that occur as you age, and explore ways to maximize your health and conditioning program with a nutritious diet.

The "fear factor"—a newly gained form of respect for horses—comes into play for the first time for many women in this age bracket. They begin to evaluate their careers, livelihood, families and physical well-being at a much higher level of priority than as a teen, and consequently may conclude that certain risks just aren't worth it. (A smaller proportion of women go in the opposite direction and begin to seek out risks.) Recognize that feeling concern or fear does not mean you're any less of a rider; it just means that you need to acknowledge and explore this new variable and its origins. As a rider, you have to take account of it and work with it. If you don't, your tension and deep-rooted fears will come through to your horse and be reflected in your reduced effectiveness as a rider.

By the time we reach our thirties, many of us have to adjust to the fact that the dream of an Olympic medal, which we have entertained since childhood, is being crowded out by more realistic goals and responsibilities. The competitive edge we've always had may have to be tempered and the psychological processes recalibrated. Some women I know have tried to keep up the same horse schedule they had in their carefree youth. They often turn around one day and realize that the schedule (not the horse) is wearing them out. Once we reduce our time commitment, the horse regains a positive and appreciated role.

Take a look at your activity and the risk factors involved. Much as you may want to fight it, making a change to a quieter horse and a more relaxed approach to riding may work best. If finding the time for riding is a problem, consider leasing a horse and sharing time with a friend to reduce stress and time commitment while still enjoying the sport. Whatever you do, don't punish yourself for some of the tradeoffs you may have to make, and don't punish an innocent horse by keeping him in circumstances where you don't have any time to do him justice.

Fit your horse, your lifestyle and your activity level into your "job description" for a successful partnership.

The Forties and Fifties

Essentially all the physical and social demands that begin to form in our twenties and thirties are usually intensified in our forties. Our bodies inevitably are beginning to show the signs of wear and tear. For example, spinal disc injuries become more prevalent due to the repeated motions of forward bending and lifting, and in most cases, sitting at a desk for inordinate amounts of time. Ligaments begin to lose elastic qualities, and it becomes more difficult to get back to optimal function. Once injuries occur, they take longer to heal.

That's the bad news. The good news is that these years can still be great physical years if you are smart about the whole picture—exercise, nutrition, preventive health care, sleep and emotional balance in your life.

This stage is when we may feel we've finally made it: job, relationships, older kids, dogs, cats, whatever, all bundled up with some leisure time and income to spend on ourselves. The balancing job is delicate, but worth it to fulfill a life dream of spending more time with your horse.

AWAREness

Most injuries that occur at this age tend to be the result of accumulated trauma and overuse, the price we pay for youthful exuberance and behaving like we are blessed with physical immortality.

To keep this dream going you must work at staying fit, healthy and nutritionally sound as well as allowing life to happen. There are going to be setbacks with horses and with the people in your immediate circle; there always are. You will need to stay open to resources, consider options and remain flexible if you and your horse pursuits are to reach true harmony.

Since more and more women in this age bracket begin to ride or pick up riding again, the forties and fifties take on particular relevance in discussing the female's biological clock and how it relates to horses.

As we enter our fourth and fifth decades, our bodies begin to dehydrate. This dehydration process results in wrinkles in our skin and decreased elasticity in our ligaments and tendons. During the mid-fifties, the intervertebral discs in our spine begin to change, becoming more spongy in character while losing the fluid-type movement that characterized our younger years. As time progresses, the vertebrae slowly begin to fuse together, limiting the spinal range of motion and decreasing the ability to accommodate compression. This is one of the reasons we literally become shorter as we age. It is also a reason why we have to be more judicious about activities that promote compression—like riding.

The major change during this phase of life is menopause. Many women experience signs of early menopause (or perimenopause) in their late thirties, and it can continue for several years. These changes include a variety of well-known symptoms. The overall effect of the changes is the decrease in estrogen, which can lead to a decrease in bone density, which can lead to osteoporosis. If osteoporosis is in your family, a thorough physical examination is recommended to reveal any areas of possible weakness in the bone mass.

Injuries that occur during these decades include ligamentous and muscular strains and tears. Some examples are shoulder rotator cuff tears and herniated discs in the spine. As with other aspects of aging, injuries take longer to heal and injured parts don't necessarily return to their former function.

Your nutrition and exercise programs are crucial to maintaining your health for riding, with particular emphasis on stretching and maintaining flexibility before placing your foot in the stirrup.

Regular exercise is essential to maintain fitness, integrity and elasticity within the ligaments and tendons of the body. Remember: What you don't use, you lose.

Over Sixty

There are no age limits to riding, but you must consider the risk factors involved and adjust your activity to suit your physical condition. In her physical therapy work, Mary Beth Walsh regularly sees patients who are in their sixties and seventies. The ones who remain active, exercise regularly, travel and have interests are in good shape and accomplish a great deal. The ones who become sedentary and sit around (sometimes in the effort to preserve themselves) deteriorate more rapidly.

AWAREness

The incidence of broken bones due to increasing brittleness and osteoporosis is a primary concern. At this age, there is a premium on common sense and judiciousness when it comes to active sports.

The mature female rider has to consider bone mass changes but should maintain an active lifestyle. The likelihood of injury has never been greater, but then neither has the reward for activity.

One thing is certain: Many gifted riders continue to ride and compete successfully well into their sixties and seventies.

Pregnancy and Riding

As a general rule, the American College of Obstetricians and Gynecologists (ACOG) states that "activities that are considered 'high risk' are not recommended during any phase of the pregnancy."

Most experienced riders don't necessarily feel that riding is a hazardous sport if they avoid certain aspects of it, such as jumping, rodeo and polo. When women ask their doctors for their recommendation on activity, most reply that you may continue any activity you performed regularly prior to your pregnancy. Put those two together and you have this finding: You can ride during pregnancy.

However, riding poses a greater risk than most sports. Simply put, you are positioned approximately six feet above ground on an unpredictable, one-thousand-pound animal. This is not what most people would consider to be safe.

Apart from the risk of falling, the jarring forces of riding can damage ligaments and joints that have slackened with your changing hormonal level. The pelvic girdle is most affected by the change in hormones. An increase in laxity in the ligaments that support it allows the bones to spread and widen the birth canal. This puts the pelvic girdle at high risk for compressive and jarring injuries that could easily be suffered with the rigors of an everyday ride.

Given these realities, we've developed a set of considerations based on the three trimesters of pregnancy. Keep in mind, however, that you can minimize but never eliminate the chances that something will go wrong. (The same can be said about virtually everything we do in life.)

In general, Mary Beth Walsh urges extreme caution during pregnancy, not only because of the inherent risks of riding but also because of the physiological changes that alter the support systems of the joints, changes in body-weight distribution that affect balance, and lung capacity issues. Damage can occur to joints due to increased laxity when abnormal compressive forces are incurred.

The decision to ride or not is a very personal one and it must be discussed with a physician. We urge you to maintain a regular exercise program, whatever you decide.

As many mothers will tell you, delivery is a major athletic event. What's more, you want to be fit to ride when it's over.

Mary Beth Walsh's Considerations on Pregnancy and Riding

The First Trimester (Months One to Three)   This is actually the most crucial period for the development of the fetus. A woman may feel nauseated and tired but not yet physically demonstrate the pregnancy. Women are encouraged to continue to exercise as long as they don't raise their core body temperature, or raise their heart rate above 140 beats per minute.

The Second Trimester (Months Three to Six)   During this phase the fetus grows in size. Physically the pregnancy presents itself, causing a protruding belly and enlarged breasts. Some women report low back pain and joint laxity, some suffer from fallen arches in their feet and many develop some sacroiliac pain as their pelvic girdle widens and the joints become more lax. Professional riders have been known to ride during this stage of pregnancy without reporting any pain or change in their riding ability. Many other women, however, report that their sense of balance is altered and their cardiovascular endurance decreases due to the pressure of the growing fetus on their lung capacity. I don't recommend riding during any phase of pregnancy, but as the fetus becomes larger, a woman's center of balance changes and endurance decreases; it places even the most experienced rider at greater risk.

The Third Trimester (Months Six to Nine)   This is the trimester for growth in size of the fetus. The larger the fetus gets, the larger the size of the mother's belly. A fetus grows from six ounces to eight to ten pounds from the fourth to the ninth month. This increase in size leads to more pressure on the lower back and decrease in lung capacity, and the hormonal changes that occur are at their maximum. Riding at this stage is extremely high-risk for everyone involved.

The following is an article I wrote for *Horse Show* magazine, the official publication of the American Horse Shows Association (AHSA). It puts in perspective the whole issue of riding and pregnancy, and just how personal a decision the choice becomes.

Riding and Pregnancy: Is It Safe?[1]

Ginny Sorkin is a professional trainer and riding instructor in Virginia and Maryland. She actively schools hunters and event horses and coaches, and her lessons and students consume most of her waking hours. When Ginny realized she was pregnant she knew there were a great deal of considerations at hand. Riding and training were her livelihood, and she wanted to continue through her pregnancy. But she asked herself, how long could she ride? Could she chance a fall? Should she stick to the ring or could she risk going on a hack?

In other words, was riding during pregnancy safe?

For Christine Culhane of Mason Neck, Virginia, riding during her pregnancies was never an issue. In fact Chris rode her normal five times per week until she had a bout with early labor. But the minute the doctor gave her permission to get back on her feet she headed for the barn and the next day delivered a healthy baby girl.

"I told the doctor I was going to ride," Christine says. "There was no discussion or choice involved. It's important to know your horse," Chris adds. "That's the key to riding or not riding while pregnant."

Dr. John Sanders, an obstetrician from Falls Church, Virginia, and an active member of the Fairfax Hunt, notes that through his experiences with pregnant riders he has seen many women that do exactly what they want to do no matter what the doctor recommends. He recalls, "There was one British woman that rode with our hunt and was a very accomplished rider; she was tough. She was my patient and I warned her of the risks but she went on anyway. She rode with the hunt up until the day she delivered. And she was only in labor for two hours."

Sanders says that riders can continue normally up until the fourth or fifth month when the pregnancy begins to show. After that you should curtail activity and cut back on any strenuous exercise. Most of all, however, Sanders advises to do what is right for you.

Riding and pregnancy. The very notion of mixing the two elicits controversy, and there are many, both within the medical profession and outside, who believe that horseback riding can endanger both horse and rider.

While there's no question that riding is good exercise, there are some hazards. But unless your pregnancy is high-risk and your doctor

[1] *Horse Show* magazine, November 1993. Reprinted by permission.

prescribes bed rest, if you are an experienced rider, chances are you can continue to ride during pregnancy for as long as it's comfortable for you to sit in the saddle.

"The main concern with riding and pregnancy is injury," states Dr. Leonard Eppard, an obstetrician from Annandale, Virginia. "There are no absolute restrictions."

Dr. Mary Vernon, a physician and medical school professor who breeds and rides Holsteiners and Lippizans, says "Most pregnant women are quite capable of sitting on a horse's back and letting the horse transport them over gentle terrain, even in the last month of pregnancy. It's probably not wise to continue jumping fences or put in a cross-country training session."

Of course, every pregnancy is unique and no rules can govern every situation. As with any kind of exercise regimen, it's imperative that pregnant riders check with their doctors before saddling up. Exercise is great for keeping unwanted weight off an expectant mom, but it's important to remember it also affects the baby. Eppard warns, "Olympic-level or exhaustive exercise can cause problems as the baby receives minimal nutrition and no fat. We have seen many growth-retarded babies due to continuous overexertion."

During intense exercise, the blood supply to the fetus can decrease. And while most women, however, will not knowingly work out hard enough to affect the baby's blood supply, it's advisable to discuss with your physician what your acceptable pulse-rate ranges and target heart rate should be.

Eppard also states that many women have a problem with fatigue in the first trimester. This certainly doesn't mix with an active lifestyle or work with what you're used to as an avid rider.

The American College of Obstetricians and Gynecologists (ACOG) advises keeping your heart rate below 140 beats per minute, but again, every pregnancy is different, so it's best to follow what your doctor recommends.

Sorkin sought out an open-minded doctor who would help her plan a pregnancy that included her equestrian lifestyle. Ultimately, she found a physician who was familiar with equestrian sports, had experience dealing with athletes, and was conveniently located to fit in with her busy schedule. After a thorough examination, he gave her the green light with the caveat that she carefully choose her mounts and not take unnecessary risks.

Peggy Cummings, a nationally recognized instructor and clinician and a speaker on the *Women & Horses* National Tour, has developed techniques which enhance body and mind awareness. She works with all levels of riders and all types of horses and has experienced pregnancy personally, with six children during her lifelong career with horses.

Peggy quips, "I remember my last pregnancy with twins because I was in the seventh month and very big. I wanted to demonstrate a movement and I mounted the horse and he groaned. I knew then it was probably best not to ride anymore."

ACOG also generally recommends avoiding jerky and bouncy movements, drinking lots of liquids before and after exercising to avoid dehydration, avoiding deep flexion or extension of joints because of the relaxation of connective tissue, avoiding strenuous exercise for more than 15 minutes and keeping up your calorie intake to reflect the exercise you're doing and baby's nutritional needs.

ACOG's guidelines are designed to accommodate active women and we can translate them for riders by suggesting that you avoid too much sitting trot and riding for long periods, especially with short stirrups.

Vernon adds that during the final trimester, the baby's position puts extra pressure on the mother's bladder. "Sitting the trot can result in wet pants," Vernon says. She suggests emptying your bladder before riding, and then for extra protection, to bring along a sanitary pad.

But each of the physicians interviewed stressed that if you are active and in good shape, you can continue to exercise, modifying intensity as you go through your pregnancy term. But if you are not active and have been fairly sedentary, do not begin exercising during pregnancy.

Pregnancy and Sports Fitness, a sports journal, advises that pregnant women should always wear protective headgear and watch for bleeding and cramps.

Physicians advise if you do experience bleeding or cramps, see your doctor right away and he or she may recommend that you curtail or stop riding and consider switching to walking or swimming. "Pain might signal something; have it checked out," Dr. Eppard notes.

The biggest concern for pregnant riders, naturally, is falling off the horse. To comply with doctor's orders meant that Ginny had to alter her teaching methods to avoid strenuous and potentially risky rides. During one cross-country clinic, for instance, where a student was having difficulty getting her horse to jump a ditch, Ginny normally would have mounted and schooled the horse herself. This time she had to stop and think. She opted not to risk it and found alternative schooling methods.

Of course, not all falls can be avoided. They happen even to the most experienced riders. Amy Hawkins, a combined training rider and mother of two, was pregnant and out for a trail ride, walking with her Thoroughbred gelding, Thistle, when he took a bad step. As the horse went down, Amy came off and hit the dirt too. Her baby was fine, but Amy ended up requiring two surgeries to fix a broken elbow. Both procedures had to be done under local anesthetic since putting her under fully would harm the baby.

One fall was enough for Amy. When she found herself pregnant with her second child, she opted to stay on the ground. She joined a health club and began a low-impact aerobic exercise class with some light weight training in place of riding.

Expectant equestrians may choose not to ride simply because it ceases to be comfortable. During pregnancy, a woman's ligaments loosen, causing hip and leg instability, which can be uncomfortable, according to Vernon. Balance shifts as well, which can also create discomfort. "Even a skilled, experienced rider may find it difficult to use her legs and seat when carrying a term fetus in her belly," Vernon says.

Cummings notes that as the baby begins to show, balance shifts. The pelvis moves forward, which causes lower back strain and pressure in the pubic area. Women can learn to release their backs and become more aware of their positions, which helps keep the pelvis freer for the job it has to perform.

If you're a tight rider, meaning you hug with your thighs and bear down into your stirrups, it will tighten your back even more and put more pressure on the baby. You will feel the weight of the baby more profoundly. The larger the baby gets, the more women tend to stand with their back arched, which causes inflammation in the back, which transfers also into her riding.

She stresses that if you feel any kind of pressure which causes strain, you should back off riding. "Women carry babies differently—some very low, some high, some toward the front, some within the body and more toward the back. This also can determine the comfort level of each rider and how she fits in the saddle," Cummings says.

Ginny rode up until her eighth month with her first child and through her seventh with her second. "It wasn't that it hurt," she recalls. "It just wasn't comfortable anymore."

Peggy Cummings recommends walking for exercise in addition or in place of riding because it is a great lower back exercise, it keeps your hips open and flexible and it helps you stay fit, which is important.

If you're like Amy and opt not to ride during pregnancy for safety reasons, or simply because it's uncomfortable, there's still plenty you can do to stay involved with your horse or barn. Ground work can be just as beneficial to your horse's training as long hours in the saddle.

You can also work with an instructor if you're not familiar with lunging and line driving. Have your instructor show you how to use a training surcingle, or thread the lines through the irons of your saddle and learn how to line drive, something you can integrate into your training program even after you deliver your baby.

Work with friends and their horses to provide them with schooling feedback from the ground. After all, you can still move a few ground poles, if you're careful. Plus, taking notes and offering comments from the sidelines can be very educational.

You can also work with a physical therapist to learn a basic massage maintenance program for your horse. Use it along with your grooming to bond with your horse and become familiar with your horse's muscle development and release points for relaxation. When you resume riding again, you may see dramatic, positive changes in your horse's attitude and performance.

You may want to consider offering services to horse people, such as blanket repair and cleaning. If you're especially creative, customize saddle pads, wraps and helmet covers or decorate tack boxes with show colors. Stay involved and keep your baby and yourself safe.

Afterword

*T*he materials in this book are the result of a lifetime with horses. I married them when I was a child, and we've been together ever since—through good times and bad, in sickness and health, for richer or poorer. And the relationship is destined to last for as long as we both shall live.

As an active lifetime rider, I entered my thirties with a buildup of physical baggage in the form of overuse and improper use. All of the years of riding and running road races culminated in a stress fracture. I suffered the fracture in my mid-back due to concussion over time, and I was laid out, immobile, for over a month. I had not been supporting my activities with a proper stretching, strengthening and weight program. I began a daily exercise program to strengthen my back and wore a rib brace for years after my injury in order to keep riding.

Then I hit thirty-nine, and thirty-nine seemed to hit back. My right shoulder became inflamed and I experienced residual neck and back pain, leading to a loss of strength. I lived with ice and ibuprofen for months, but couldn't continue on like that forever. On examination, my doctor identified a tear in my rotator cuff. This was attributed, once again, to overuse and improper use, and lack of preparation for my sport. I am five feet four inches, and I've spent a lifetime reaching up to work with horses, always using my right side. With a little more forethought, preparation and prevention, I probably could have avoided the surgery that cost me months of riding time and enjoyment.

No major accidents, just lack of understanding about my body in general and my body on horseback in particular. The most frustrating part, now that I look back, is that little of the information we have imparted in this book was available or included in my years of riding education. I couldn't have known it—couldn't have prevented some of the problems—even if I had wanted to. You just groomed, tacked and rode, without a basic understanding of *your* body or knowledge of how to stop bad things (*unnecessary* bad things) from happening.

Based on those experiences, I learned a few things. Riding isn't just about strength. And it's not just about pushing the right buttons on your horse. Yet nothing I had learned in thirty-five years of riding and formal "classical" training seemed to hold the answers. The issue was bigger than me—it involved an entire class of riders, modern female riders, for whom the foundations, concepts and techniques of bygone eras were no longer adequate.

I took on a project to regroup, personally and professionally. Through relationships over the past few years with many wonderful professionals, including the contributors to this book, I have come to understand that, when it comes to riding, the issues of form and fitness have their own particular female side—a side which, until now, had yet to be fully and forcefully articulated.

I began to put it all together.

The key to good riding is to understand your body, your horse's body and the way the two interact. Along the way, you have to listen, feel, touch. The people best equipped to do that, for a variety of innate and societal reasons, are women. Allowed to pursue her own intuitions and methods, the human female can achieve superior results and a world of gratification from her horse.

With that knowledge in place, another barrier presents itself: Traditions governing riding instruction and equipment remain male-oriented and, for that reason, outdated. The dramatic rise in female participation in horse activities in the late twentieth century has not, to date, been matched by a commensurate amount of rethinking of the methods and materials used to train a horse.

These two areas come together in the process that this book introduces: *a way of looking at, thinking about, preparing for and executing female-oriented riding.* And this is just the beginning. Young women make up 90 percent of the enrollment in college-level riding programs and probably

95 percent of the participants in weekend shows across the country. That is the future of horse*man*ship!

In my first Women & Horses Workshop, out of 200 attendees, only a few women were able to raise their hands to indicate they were healthy, injury-free riders. The rest of us identified with chronic back or neck pain, shoulder pain, or strength issues. And that was *before* we discussed the demands of time, family, money, lifestyle, and so on. In my travels since, I have seen to an even greater degree how our life issues and our horse issues cross paths.

Putting it all together. Realizing the greatest possible return from your experience with horses.

I believe this book can be the departure point in your effort to "put it all together" and realize the greatest possible return from your experience with horses. I hope you'll share your experiences with me (and anyone else who will listen).

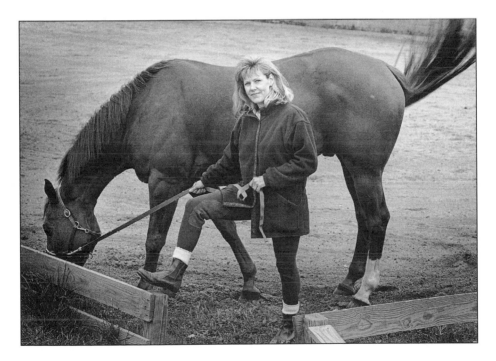

Bibliography

Allen, John. *Principles of Modern Riding for Ladies.* London: R. Griffin & Co., 1825.

The American Heart Association. "An Eating Plan for Healthy Americans," National Center, Dallas, Texas. Eating Right with Dietary Guidelines - U.S.D.A., U.S. H.H.S., and F.M.I. Washington, D.C., 1991.

Apsley, Lady, and Lady Diane Shedden. *"To Whom the Goddess." Riding and Hunting for Women.* London: Hutchinson & Co., 1932.

Beach, Belle. *Riding & Driving for Women.* New York: Charles Scribner's Sons, 1912.

Benardot, D. *Sports Nutrition—A Guide for the Professional Working with Active People,* Sports and Cardiovascular Nutritionists (SCAN), Practice Group of The American Dietetic Association. Chicago: The American Dietetic Association Publication, 1993.

Bennett, Deborah. "Who Is Built Best to Ride?" *Equus,* volume 140 (1989): 58–64.

Bernardi, C. *Sports Nutrition: Strategies for Success, Energy and Fluid Needs For Athletes,* Georgetown R.D. Outpatient Nutrition Services Sports Program. Washington, D.C.: Georgetown University Hospital, 1993.

Berning, J. S., and N. Steen. *Sports Nutrition for the 90's— The Health Professional's Handbook.* Gaithersburg, Md.: ASPEN Publications, 1991.

Christy, Eva. *Modern Side-Saddle Riding.* London: Vinton & Co. Ltd., 1907.

Clark, N. *How to Eat to Win—The Athlete's Kitchen.* New York: Bantam Books, 1981.

Clark, N. *Nancy Clark's Sports Nutrition Guidebook—Eating to Fuel Your Active Lifestyle.* Champaign, Ill.: Leisure Press, 1990.

Clarke, Stirling J. *The Habit & The Horse: A Treatis on Female Equitation.* London: Smith, Elder & Co., 1857.

Davies, George, and James Gould. *Orthopaedic and Sports Physical Therapy.* St. Louis: The C. V. Mosby Co., 1985.

DeHurst, C. *How Women Should Ride.* New York: Harper & Bros, 1892.

Diggle, Martin. *Teaching the Mature Rider.* London: J. A. Allen & Co., 1993.

Goldschmidt, S. G. Lt. Col. *The Fellowship of the Horse.* New York: Charles Scribner's Sons, 1930.

Gottschlich, M. M., L. E. Matarese, and E .P. Shronts. *Nutrition Support Dietetics-Core Curriculum,* American Society For Parenteral & Enteral Nutrition. Silver Spring, Md.: A.S.P.E.N. Publications, 1993.

Karr, Elizabeth. *The American Horsewoman.* Boston: Houghton, Mifflin & Co., 1884.

Kendall, Florence, and Elizabeth McCreary. *Muscles Testing and Function,* 4th ed. Baltimore: Williams & Wilkins Co., 1983.

Kotsonis, F. N., and M. A. Mackey. *Nutrition in the "90s": Current Controversies and Analysis,* vol. 2, New York: Marcel Dekker, Inc., 1994.

Magee, David J. *Orthopaedic Physical Assessment.* Philadelphia: W. B. Saunders Co., 1987.

McArdle, William, Frank I. Katch, and Victor L. Katch. *Exercise Physiology, Energy, Nutrition and Human Performance,* 2nd ed. Philadelphia: Lea & Febiger, 1986.

McArdle, W. D., F. I. Katch, and V. L. Katch. *Exercise Physiology,* 3rd ed. Philadelphia: Lea & Febiger, 1991.

Meyners, Eckhart. *Fit for Riding.* Middleton, Md.: Half Halt Press, 1986.

Mittlemark, Raul Artal, M.D., and Robert A. Wiswell. *Exercise in Pregnancy*. Baltimore: Williams & Wilkens Publishing Co., 1986.

Moore, Keith L. *Clinically Oriented Anatomy*. Baltimore: Williams & Wilkens Publishing Co., 1985.

Myers, Michael. "Practical Horseman," *Back in Shape* 21, no. 4 (April 1993): 44–50, 96.

Nash, J. D. *Maximize Your Body Potential*. Palo Alto, Calif.: Bull Publishing Co., 1986.

O'Donoghue, (Mrs.) Power. *Riding for Ladies*. London: W. Thacker and Company, 1887.

Peterson, M., and K. Peterson. *Eat to Compete: A Guide to Sports Nutrition*. Chicago: Year Book Medical Publishers, Inc., 1988.

Saunders, Duane H. *Evaluation, Treatment and Prevention of Muscoskeletal Disorders*. Minneapolis: Anderburg-Lund Printing Company, 1986.

Schusdziarra H., and V. Schudziarra. *The Anatomy of a Rider*. Briarcliff, N.Y.: Breakthrough Publications, 1978.

Skelton, Betty. *Side Saddle Riding*. London: The Sportsman's Press, 1988.

Soderburg, Gary L. *Kinesiology, Application to Pathological Motion*. Baltimore: Williams & Wilkens Publishing Company, 1986.

Stanley, Edward. *The Young Horsewoman's Compendium of the Modern Art of Riding*. London: James Ridgeway, 1827.

Contributors

Peggy Cummings
Equestrian Clinician and Trainer, Hailey, Idaho

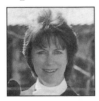 Peggy Cummings, an internationally recognized equitation specialist, has been involved with horses her entire life. She began riding as a child in El Salvador and later moved to Maine. She taught at a girls' camp for many years and also instructed in Pony Club.

After years of competing and training, Peggy owned and managed her own training stable and launched her career as a professional instructor, clinician, and trainer. She travels extensively conducting clinics in her methods and techniques, which have become an integral and successful part of many riding programs.

She holds numerous certifications, among them Centered Riding Master Instructor and T.T.E.A.M. Practitioner, Horsemaster, and has received training from the United States Dressage Federation Instructors' Clinics and the American Dressage Institute.

Peggy has been featured in presentations before the American Endurance Riding Conference, United States Pony Clubs, 4-H, the United States Equestrian Team, All-American Quarter Horse Congress, and the North American Riding for the Handicapped Association. Her clinics include, but are not limited to instructor education, customized saddle fitting, stress reduction and awareness for professional people on the go, and handicapped and youth programs.

Peggy is a Women & Horses Workshop and National Tour expert and presenter.

Mary Beth Walsh, P.T., Dip. M.D.T.
Marymount University, Arlington, Virginia

Mary Beth Walsh is a physical therapist on faculty with the Physical Therapy program at Marymount University in Arlington, Virginia. She has combined her British Horse Society Assistant Instructor Certification and experience as a physical therapist to evaluate equestrian biomechanics and orthopedic injury.

She received her bachelor of science degree in Physical Therapy at New York University in 1988. She received postgraduate certification in Mechanical Diagnosis and Treatment from the McKenzie Institute in Wellington, New Zealand, in 1992, and is currently working toward a master of arts degree in Education from The George Washington University in Washington, D.C., with a subspeciality in public health administration. She is licensed to practice in the District of Columbia and Virginia.

Her physical therapy practice is in Orthopedic Sports Medicine, specializing in the treatment of the spine. She has developed a comprehensive equestrian rehabilitation program based in northern Virginia. She has also worked with neurologically involved riders through the "Lift Me Up" program in Great Falls, Virginia.

Mary Beth published an article in 1991 for the *Advance for Physical Therapists* magazine titled, "Therapist Prepares Equestrians for Safe, Effective Riding."

Mary Beth Walsh is a Women & Horses Workshop and National Tour expert and presenter.

Margaret M. McGovern, MBA, R.D., L.D.
Licensed Nutrition Consultant, Silver Spring, Maryland

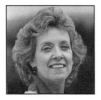

Margaret (Peg) M. McGovern, MBA, is a licensed and registered dietitian currently providing nutrition services in private practice in the Washington, D.C. area and in Maryland. She served as assistant director of Food and Nutrition Services at the Georgetown University Medical Center in Washington, D.C., for over ten years. She also provided clinical nutrition education to in- and out-patients at G.U. Medical Center for over twenty years.

Peg received her undergraduate bachelor of science degree from Duchesne College in Omaha, Nebraska, and her master of Business Administration degree from Marymount University in Arlington, Virginia. She is a licensed dietitian in Washington, D.C., and in the State of Maryland, and a registered dietitian nationally.

She has served as chairperson and committee member of Georgetown University Medical Center's Annual Nutrition Services Symposium and is a member of The American Heart Association's Nutrition Symposium.

Acknowledgments

Special thanks to

- Tom Aronson, my husband, business associate and best friend. His love and his wisdom are my foundation for living.

- Jane Midkiff Polk, my mother, for her deep love, always setting an example as a leader in her career and in the community, for her guidance as I grew up, and for reminding me to strive to become not only the best woman, but more importantly, the best person. And to her husband and my step-father, Reed, who has always supported me unconditionally.

- Dan B. Midkiff, Jr., my father, for his common sense and gentle nature, and for passing on his love of the land to me. And my grandfather, Dan B. Midkiff, Sr., who loved horses as much as I do. It was from this side of the family that I received the "horse gene."

- Dan B. Midkiff, III, my brother, for putting up with a horse-crazy sister for the past forty years.

- Contributing writers Mary Beth Walsh, P.T.; Peggy Cummings; and Peg McGovern. Their input and expertise have made this book possible.

- Horse thanks to our "cover boy" Horton (Critical Mass), Tarim, Kippy's Surprise, and Whiz Kid for modeling in the book.

And to many others who assisted in making this book possible:

Howard Allen; Sharon Anthony; Ariat; Virginia Artho, National Cowgirl Hall of Fame; Paul Belton, Albion Saddlemakers; Dr. Deb Bennett, Equine Studies Institute; Dr. Chongwen Cai, Dr. Chen Yong and Wei Ping, Sports Injury Therapy Clinic; Anne Calligan; Alix Coleman, photographer; Susan Cook; Gwyn Donohue; Gwen Edsall, equine muscle therapist; Rich Frazier, photographer;

Amy Gill; Steve Ray Gonzalez, SR Saddlery; Penny Goring, *Dressage* magazine; Dawn Haney, illustrator; Jan Jacobson, Performance Saddlery; Helen Junkin; Markel Insurance Co.; Tom and Alice Magaha, Hedgeland Farm; Sue Mandas; Joan Peyton; Julie Podolny, Equi-Logic; William Poehler, Tack 'n Togs Merchandising; Liz and Ralph Potter; Laura Rose and Peter Winants, National Sporting Library; Sun Valley Herb Company; Chrystine Tauber, USET; Dr. Rick Timms, Troxel; Christina Van Houdt, Support Team; Dr. Mary Vernon; Donna Walker, physical therapist; Ellen Wessel, Moving Comfort; Jennifer Wofford; and Leslie Wood, instructor.

Much love and thanks to our dog Boomer, a crucial part of my life support system.

And lastly, thanks to all of the horses with which I have shared experiences. They continue to offer fascinating and meaningful insights into my life and remain the key to my bliss.

This book is in memory of Margaret Watters for her unwavering love and dedication to horses and their quality of life.

Index